Frequently Asked Questions
OPERATIVE DENTISTRY AND ENDODONTICS

Frequently Asked Questions

OPERATIVE DENTISTRY AND ENDODONTICS

*A free companion to
Essential Quick Review:
Operative Dentistry and Endodontics*

Editor-in-Chief

Priya Verma Gupta MDS FPFA
Professor
Department of Pedodontics and Preventive Dentistry
Divya Jyoti College of Dental Sciences and Research
Ghaziabad, Uttar Pradesh, India

Co-Author

Vivek Hegde BDS MDS
Vice Principal, Professor and Head of the Department
Department of Operative Dentistry and Endodontics
M.A. Rangoonwala Dental College
Pune, Maharashtra, India

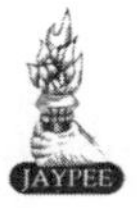

The Health Sciences Publisher

New Delhi | London | Philadelphia | Panama

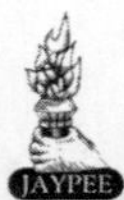

Jaypee Brothers Medical Publishers (P) Ltd

Headquarters
Jaypee Brothers Medical Publishers (P) Ltd
4838/24, Ansari Road, Daryaganj
New Delhi 110 002, India
Phone: +91-11-43574357
Fax: +91-11-43574314
Email: jaypee@jaypeebrothers.com

Overseas Offices

J.P. Medical Ltd
83 Victoria Street, London
SW1H 0HW (UK)
Phone: +44 20 3170 8910
Fax: +44 (0)20 3008 6180
Email: info@jpmedpub.com

Jaypee-Highlights Medical Publishers Inc.
City of Knowledge, Bld. 235, Clayton
Panama City, Panama
Phone: +1 507-301-0496
Fax: +1 507-301-0499
Email: cservice@jphmedical.com

Jaypee Medical Inc.
325 Chestnut Street
Suite 412, Philadelphia,
PA 19106, USA
Phone: +1 267-519-9789
Email: support@jpmedus.com

Jaypee Brothers Medical Publishers (P) Ltd
17/1-B Babar Road, Block-B, Shaymali
Mohammadpur, Dhaka-1207
Bangladesh
Mobile: +08801912003485
Email: jaypeedhaka@gmail.com

Jaypee Brothers Medical Publishers (P) Ltd
Bhotahity, Kathmandu, Nepal
Phone: +977-9741283608
Email: kathmandu@jaypeebrothers.com

Website: www.jaypeebrothers.com
Website: www.jaypeedigital.com

Inquiries for bulk sales may be solicited at: jaypee@jaypeebrothers.com

Frequently Asked Questions: Operative Dentistry and Endodontics

First Edition: **2016**

ISBN: 978-93-86107-81-7

Printed at Rajkamal Electric Press, Plot No. 2, Phase-IV, Kundli, Haryana.

Editorial Board

Preface

I am very pleased to introduce you to the first edition of Essential Quick Review; A series for final year undergraduate students.

The series will be available in eight subjects, i.e., Periodontics, Operative Dentistry and Endodontics, Pedodontics, Prosthodontics, Oral Surgery, Oral Medicine and Radiology, Orthodontics and Public Health Dentistry covering essential parts of each subject. This book will not only help the student to attain the knowledge, but will also give an idea how to attempt a question during the examination, covering entire syllabus in a limited period of time.

It is a supplementary booklet for each subject that contains three sections, i.e., definitions, classifications and viva-voce covering the entire syllabus enabling the student to undergo a quick revision. The language used is very simple for better understanding.

The study material provided in this book is an attempt to provide an additional help to students for easy retention and reproduction of subject in the examination. This book is in no way a replacement to standard text book.

I thank all my subject matter experts for their valued suggestions and contributions. A very special word of thanks to my family for being the source of constant encouragement.

I profusely thank Shri Jitendar P Vij (CEO), Mr Ankit Vij (Group President), and production team of M/S Jaypee Brothers Medical Publishers (P) Ltd, New Delhi for their enthusiasm and constant efforts in bringing out this book.

Priya Verma Gupta

Contents

1. Definitions 1-24

2. Classifications 25-48

3. Viva-Voce 49-112

Definitions

Endodontics

It is the branch of clinical dentistry associated with the prevention, diagnosis and treatment of pathosis of the dental pulp and their sequelae. Thus, the main aim of the endodontic therapy involves to: maintain vitality of the pulp, preserve and restore the teeth which have failed to the previous endodontic therapy, including those with damaged and necrotic pulp. Endo is a Greek word for "Inside" and Odont is Greek word for "Tooth". Endodontic treatment deals inside of the tooth.

Endodontist

An endodontist is a dentist who undergoes a special training in diagnosing and treating the problems associated with inside of the tooth.

Dental pulp

The dental pulp is soft tissue of mesenchymal origin located in center of a tooth. It consists of specialized cells, odontoblasts arranged peripherally in direct contact with dentin matrix. This close relationship between odontoblasts and dentin is known as pulp-dentin complex. It is surrounded by rigid walls and so is unable to expand in response to injury. The various zones of pulp are: odontoblastic layer at the pulp periphery, cell free zone of weil, cell rich zone and pulp core.

Odontoblasts

Cells originating from neural crest with the biologic function of formation of dentin. These cells synthesize mainly type. I collagen and proteoglycans with a morphology that reflects their functional activity. Their number ranges from 59,000–76,000/mm^2 in coronal dentin, usually lesser in root dentin.

Pulp chamber

The pulp cavity portion present in the crown of tooth. It reflects the external form of enamel at the time of eruption, but anatomy is less sharply defined. The roof of pulp chamber consists of dentin covering the pulp chamber occlusally.

Canal orifices

These are openings in the floor of pulp chamber leading into the root canals.

Root canal

It is that portion of pulp cavity which extends from canal orifice to the apical foramen. The shape of root canal varies with size, shape and number of the roots in different teeth.

Apical foramen

It is an aperture at or near the apex of a root through which nerves and blood vessels of the pulp enter or leave the pulp cavity. Normally, it is present near the apex but sometimes, opening may be present on the accessory and lateral canals of root surface forming the accessory foramina.

Pulp stones/denticles

Pulp stones are nodular,calcified masses appearing in either coronal and radicular pulp or both of them. The larger calcifications are called denticles. It is seen that pulp stones are present in at least 50 percent of teeth. Pulp stones may either occur as a natural phenomenon or due to some injury.

Cementum

The hard, avascular connective tissue that covers the roots of the teeth and is formed by cells known as cementoblasts. It is light yellow in color and can be differentiated from enamel by its darker hue and lack of luster, although it is slightly lighter in color than dentin. It is highly permeable to dyes and various chemical agents.

Periodontal ligament

Periodontal ligament is a unique,complex connective tissue structure that provides a continous adapting apparatus between alveolar bone and cementum. It is continuous with connective tissue of the gingiva and communicates with the marrow spaces through vascular channels in the bone. It houses the fibers, particularly collagen, numerous cells, blood vessels nerves and an extracellular substance with variety of polysaccharides and proteins.

Periodontal fibers

The most important component of periodontal ligament are principal fibers. These fibers are composed mainly of collagen Type I. Apart from the principal fibers, oxytalan and elastic fibers are also present. The principal fibers are present in six different types of arrangements.

Horizontal group

These fibers are arranged horizontally at right angles re-stricted to coronal half of periodontal ligament originating from cementum and attached to the alveolar bone.

Alveolar crest group

These fibers arise from cementum in fan like manner and attach to the alveolar crest. These fibers prevent the lateral tooth movement and extrusion.

Oblique fibers

These fibers make the largest group in periodontal ligament. They extend from cementum to bone obliquely. They bear the occlusal forces and transmit them to alveolar bone.

Transseptal fibers

These fibers run from cementum of one tooth to the cementum of another tooth crossing over the alveolar crest.

Apical fibers

These fibers are arranged irregularly, radiating from cementum to bone present around the root apex.

Interradicular fibers

These fibers are present in furcation areas of multirooted teeth extending from inter-radicular septum.

Nerve fibers

The nerve fibers present in periodontal ligament, are either of myelinated or non-myelinated type.

Blood vessels

The periodontal ligament receives blood supply from the gingival, alveolar and apical vessels.

Alveolar bone

Bone is specialized connective tissue which comprises of thin, compact bone that forms and supports the sockets which surround the tooth root.

Irreversible pulpitis

It is a persistent inflammatory condition of the pulp, symptomatic or asymptomatic, caused by a noxious stimulus. It has both acute and chronic stages in pulp.

Chronic pulpitis

It is an inflammatory response of pulpal connective tissue to an irritant, pain is absent because of diminished exudative inflammatory activity and corresponding decrease in intrapulpal pressure to a point below threshold limits of pain receptors. Chronic pulpitis can be of three types: ulcerative/open form, hyperplastic form and closed form.

Pulp necrosis

Pulp necrosis is a condition following untreated pulpitis. The pulpal tissue becomes dead and if the condition is not treated, noxious materials will leak from pulp space forming the lesion of endodontic origin.

Pulp degeneration

Pulp degeneration is generally found in old age. It may be the result of persistent mild irritation in young age. Usually, it is induced by attrition, abrasion, erosion, bacteria, operative procedures, caries, pulp capping and reversible pulpitis.

Acute apical periodontitis

Painful inflammation of the periodontium as a result of trauma, irritation or infection through the root canal, regardless of whether the pulp is vital or nonvital. It is an inflammation around the apex of a tooth. The distinctive features of acute apical periodontitis (AAP) are microscopic rather than roentogenographic, symptomatic rather than visible.

Acute apical abscess

It is a localized collection of pus in the alveolar bone at the root apex of the tooth, following the death of pulp with extension of the infection through the apical foramen into periradicular tissue.

Phoenix abscess/recrudescent abscess

An acute inflammatory reaction superimposed on an existing chronic lesion, such as a cyst or granuloma. In other words, phoenix abscess is an acute exacerbation of a chronic lesion.

Periapical granuloma

Periapical granuloma is one of the most common sequelae of pulpitis. It is usually described as a mass of chronically inflamed granulation tissue found at the apex of nonvital tooth.

Radicular cyst

The radicular cyst is an inflammatory cyst which results because of extension of infection from pulp into the surrounding periapical tissues.

Chronic alveolar abscess

Chronic alveolar abscess is also known as suppurative apical periodontitis which is associated with gradual egress of irritants from root canal system into periradicular area leading to formation of an exudate.

Persistent apical periodontitis

It is post-treatment apical periodontitis in an endodontically treated tooth. *Enterococcus faecalis* is found most consistently reported organism in persistent apical periodontitis.

External root resorption

Resorption is a condition associated with either physiologic or pathologic process that results in loss of substance from tissues like dentin, cementum or alveolar bone. In external root resorption, root resorption affects the cementum or dentin of the root. It can be: apical, lateral and cervical.

Anachoresis

Anachoresis refers to the attraction of blood borne bacteria in the areas of inflammation. It is a process by which microorganisms are transported in the blood to an area of inflammation where they cause an infection.

Biofilm

A sessile, multi-cellular, microbial community characterized by cells that are firmly attached to a surface and enmeshed in a self produced matrix of extracellular polymeric substances. Various types of endodontic biofilms are: intracanal, extraradicular and periapical.

Photoactivated disinfection

It is a combination of a photosensitizer solution and low-power laser light. Photodynamic therapy/light activated therapy destroys an endodontic biofilm when a photo-sensitizer selectively accumulated in the target cell is activated, by a visible light of appropriate wavelength.

Inflammation

Inflammation is defined as the local response of living mammalian tissue to injury.

Signs of inflammation

The roman writer Celsus in 1st century AD gave four cardinal signs of inflammation: rubor (redness), tumor (swelling), color (heat) and dolor (pain).

Diagnosis

It is defined as utilization of scientific knowledge for identifying a diseased process and to differentiate it from other disease processes. In other words, literal meaning of diagnosis is determination and judgment of variations from the normal.

Case history

The purpose of case history is to discover whether patient has any general or local condition that might alter the normal course of treatment.

Chief complaint

It consists of information which promoted patient to visit a clinician. Phenomenon symptoms or signs of deviation from normal are indicative of illness.

Symptoms

Symptoms are defined as signs of departure from the normal. They are indicators of illness.

Pulp Oximetry

A noninvasive device for determining pulp vitality. The principle of this technology is based on modification of Beer's law and the absorbency characteristics of hemoglobin in red and infrared range.

Plethysmography

It is a method for assessing the changes in volume and has been applied to the investigation of arterial disease because the volume of the limb or organ exhibits transient changes over the cardiac cycle.

Digital radiography

Digital imaging uses standard radiology techniques with film to record the image.It then subjects the finished image to digital processing to produce the final image.

Digital dental radiology

Images in digital form can be readily manipulated, stored and retrieved on computer. Furthermore, this technology helps to make the transmission of images practicable.

Cleaning

It is the process which physically removes contamination but does not necessarily destroy microorganisms. It is a prerequisite before decontamination by disinfection or sterilization of instruments since organic material prevents contact with microbes, inactivates disinfectants.

Disinfection

It is the process of using an agent that destroys germs or other harmful microbes or inactivates them, usually it refers to chemicals that kill the vegetative forms but not the resistant spores of bacteria.

Antisepsis

It is the destruction of pathogenic microorganisms existing in their vegetative state on living tissues.

Sterilization

Sterilization involves any process, physical or chemical, that will destroy all forms of life, including bacterial, fungi, spores and viruses.

Aseptic technique

It is the method which prevents contamination of wounds and other sites, by ensuring that only sterile objects and fluids come into contact with them; so that the risks of airborne contamination are minimized.

Antiseptic

It is a chemical applied to living tissues, such as skin or mucous membrane to reduce the number of microorganisms present, either by inhibition of their activity or by destroying them.

Disinfectant

It is a chemical substance, which causes disinfection. It is used on nonvital objects to kill surface vegetative pathogenic organisms, but not necessarily spore forms or viruses.

Pulp cavity

The pulp cavity lies within the tooth and is enclosed by dentin all around, except at the apical foramen. It is divided into two parts; coronal and radicular.

Pulp horns

These are landmarks present occlusal to pulp chamber. They may vary in height and location, tends to be single horn associated with each cusp of posterior teeth and mesial and distal in anterior teeth.

Canal orifice

Canal orifices are openings in the floor of pulp chamber leading into root canals.

Gemination

It arises from an attempt at division of a single tooth germ by an invagination resulting in incomplete formation of two teeth.

Fusion

Fusion results in union two normally separated tooth germ. Fused teeth may show separate or fused pulp space.

Concrescence

The type of fusion in which teeth are joined by cementum only, after the root formation has completed.

Taurodontism

In this, body of tooth is enlarged at the expense of roots (also called bull like teeth). Pulp chamber of this tooth is extremely large with a greater apico-occlusal height .Bifurcation/trifurcation may be present only few millimeters above the root apex. Pulp lacks the normal constriction at cervical level of tooth.This condition is commonly seen associated with syndromes like Klinefelter syndrome and Down syndrome.

Talon's cusp

It resembles eagle's talon. In this, anamolous structure projects lingually from the cingulum area of maxillary or mandibular incisor. This structure blends smoothly with the tooth except that there is a deep developmental groove where that structure blends with lingual surface of the tooth.

Dilaceration

Dilaceration is an extraordinary curving of the roots of the teeth. Its etiology is usually related to trauma during the root development in which movement of the crown and a part of root may result in sharp angulation after tooth completes development.

Dentinogenesis imperfecta

An autosomal dominant development disturbance of dentin that affects both permanent as well as the deciduous dentition.Grey to yellowish-brown tooth with broad crown constricting at the cervical portion resembling a tulip is the characterisitic feature.

Dentin dysplasia

It is rare disturbance, characterized by formation of normal enamel, atypical dentin with abnormal pulpal morphology.

In this,involved tooth appears normal clinically, but root canals are usually obliterated so require special care during instrumentation. It is known as rootless teeth and can affect both dentitions.

Dens in dente or dens invaginatus

This developmental variation represents an accentuation lingually, that occurs in the surface of crown of tooth before calcification due to various postulated reasons,such as, focal growth stimulation or retardation,increase in external pressure in different parts of tooth bud. The most commonly involved tooth is maxillary lateral incisor.

Dens evaginatus

In this development condition, an anomalous tubercle or accessory cusp is located on the occlusal surface bilaterally or unilaterally in between lingual and buccal cusps. Due to occlusal abrasion, this tubercle wears off fast causing early exposure of accessory pulp horn that extends into the tubercle. This may further result in periradicular pathology in otherwise caries free teeth even before completion of the apical root development. This condition is commonly seen in premolars, while rarely, incisors,cuspids and molars.

Access cavity preparation

An endodontic coronal preparation which enables unobstructed access to the canal orifices, a straight line access to apical foramen, complete control over instrumentation and accommodate obturation technique.

EDTA

It is relatively nontoxic and slightly irritating in weak solutions. The effect of this on dentin depends on the concentration of it's solution and length of contact time with dentin.

Apical foramen

The main apical opening of the root canal which may be located away from anatomic or radiographic apex.

Apical constriction

It is apical portion of root canal having narrowest diameter. It is usually 0.5–1 mm short of apical foramen.

Cementodentinal junction

The region where cementum and dentin are united, the point at which cemental surface terminates at or near the apex of tooth. It is not always necessary that cementodentinal junction always coincide with apical constriction.

Cleaning

It comprises various steps involved in the removal of all potentially pathogenic content from the root canals of tooth.

Shaping

The establishment of a specifically shaped cavity which performs the dual role of three-dimensional progressive access into the canal and creating an apical preparation which will permit easy manipulation of final materials and obturation instruments.

Dentin chip filling

In this technique, after through cleaning and shaping of canal, H-file is used to produce dentin powder in central portion of the canal, which is then packed apically with butt end of paper point. It forms a biologic seal.

Single visit endodontics (SVE)

It implies to cleaning, shaping and disinfection of a root canal system followed by obturation of the root canal during the same appointment.

Endodontic emergency

The condition associated with pain and/or swelling which requires immediate diagnosis and treatment. The main causative factors responsible for occurrence of endodontic emergencies are pathosis and traumatic injuries in pulp and periradicular tissues. These are categorized into three main types: pretreatment, intra-appointment and postobturation.

Cracked tooth syndrome

The crack tooth syndrome means incomplete fracture of a tooth with vital pulp. The fracture commonly involves enamel and dentin but sometimes pulp and periodontal structure may also get involved. It is commonly seen to be associated in teeth with large and complex restorations.

Acute reversible pulpitis

This condition is characterized by localized inflammation of the pulp, lowering of threshold stimulation for α-delta nerve fibers, exaggerated and nonlingering response to stimuli.

Acute irreversible pulpitis

It is characterized by presence of inflammatory mediators which lower the threshold of stimulation, for all intrapulpal nerves. There is a history of spontaneous pain and exaggerated response to hot or cold that lingers even after the stimulus is removed. Extensive restoration or caries may be seen in the involved tooth and lingering pain occurs after thermal stimulation of α-delta nerve fibers while spontaneous dull, aching pain occurs by stimulation of unmyelinated C-fibers in the pulp.

Acute periapical abscess

It is a collection of pus, usually caused by an infection that has spread from tooth to the surrounding tissues.

Acute apical periodontitis

It is an inflammation of periodontal ligament caused by tissue damage usually from extension of pulpal pathosis or occlusal trauma. It is characterized by elevation of tooth out of its socket due to build up in fluid pressure in the periodontal ligament. The patient complaint of discomfort in biting or chewing and sensitivity to percussion is a hallmark test for its diagnosis.

Tissue emphysema

It is defined as collection of gas or air in the tissue spaces or facial planes.

Healing

It is a dynamic process, reduced radiolucency combined with normal clinical presentation.

Disease

No change or increase in radiolucency, clinical signs may or may not be present or vice versa.

Canal blockage

A blockage is obstruction in a previously patent canal system that prevents access to the apical constriction or apical stop.

Ledge

Ledge is an internal transportation of the canal which prevents positioning of an instrument to the apex in an otherwise patent canal.

Apical Canal transportation

The change in position of canal's normal anatomic foramen to a new location on external root surface.

Overinstrumentation

The excessive instrumentation beyond the apical constriction violates the periodontal ligament and alveolar bone.

Overpreparation

It is excessive removal of tooth structure in mesiodistal and buccolingual direction.

Underpreparation

It is the failure to remove pulp tissue, dentinal debris and microorganisms from the root canal system.

Perforation

The mechanical or pathological communication between the root canal system and the external tooth surface.

Endodontic surgery

The removal of tissues other than the contents of root canal to retain a tooth with pulpal or periapical involvement.

Full mucoperiosteal flaps

In this procedure, the entire soft tissue overlying the cortical plate in the surgical site is reflected.

Trapezoidal flap

It is formed by two releasing incisions which join a horizontal intrasulcular incision at obtuse angles. It was described by Neumann and Eikan in 1940.

Replantation

The act of deliberately removing a tooth and following examination, diagnosis, endodontic manipulation and repair–returning the tooth to its original socket. It was defined by Grossman in 1982. It can be of two types, intentional and unintentional.

Transplantation

It is the procedure of replacement of a tooth in a socket other than the one from which it had been extracted from.

Suturing

The procedure which is used to approximate incised tissues and also stabilize the flapped mucoperiosteum until reattachment occurs. A suture is strand of material used to close the wound.

Extraoral ecchymosis (extraoral discoloration)

Discoloration/ecchymosis usually results when blood has leaked into the surrounding tissues. This condition is self limiting in nature and lasts up to 2 weeks and does not affect the prognosis.

Endo-perio lesions

An endo-perio lesion is one where both pulp and periodontal tissues are affected by the disease progress.

Crown infraction

A crown infraction is incomplete fracture of enamel without loss of tooth structure. This type of injury is very common but often unnoticed. It results from traumatic impact to enamel and appears as craze line running parallel with direction of enamel rods and ending at dentinoenamel junction.

Uncomplicated crown fracture

Crown fracture involving enamel and dentin not pulp is called uncomplicated crown fracture.

Complicated crown fracture

Crown fracture involving enamel, dentin and pulp is called complicated crown fracture.

Pulp capping

Pulp capping implies placing the dressing directly onto the pulp exposure.

Pulpotomy

Pulpotomy refers only to coronal extirpation of vital pulp tissue. It is of two types partial and full (cervical).

Cervical pulpotomy/deep pulpotomy

Cervical pulpotomy involves removal of entire coronal pulp to the level of root orifices.

Apexification

The process which stimulates formation of a calcified barrier across the apex particularly, in an immature tooth, if pulp tissue is necrotic.

Crown root fracture

Crown root fracture involves enamel, dentin and cementum with or without the involvement of pulp. It is usually oblique in nature involving both crown and root. This type of injury is considered as more complex type of injury because of its greater severity and involvement of the pulp.

Root fracture

These are uncommon injuries but represent a complex healing pattern due to involvement of dentin, cementum, pulp and periodontal ligament.

Luxation injuries

Luxation injuries cause trauma to supporting structures of teeth ranging from minor crushing of periodontal ligament and neurovascular supply of pulp to total displacement of the teeth. They are usually caused by sudden impact such as blow, fall or striking a hard object.

Subluxation

An injury to the tooth supporting structures resulting in increased mobility, but without displacement of the tooth. Teeth are sensitive to percussion and have some mobility. Sulcular bleeding is seen showing damage and rupture of the periodontal ligament fibers. Pulp responds normal to testing. Tooth is not displaced.

Lateral luxation

In lateral luxation, trauma displaces the tooth lingually, buccally, mesially or distally, in other words, out of its normal position away from its long axis. Sulcular bleeding is present indicating rupture of periodontal ligament fibers. Tooth is sensitive to percussion. Clinically, crown of laterally luxated tooth is usually displaced horizontally with tooth locked firmly in the new position, percussion may elicit metallic tone indicating that root has forced into the alveolar bone.

Extrusive luxation

In extrusive luxation, tooth is displaced from the socket along its long axis, tooth is very mobile with the visible displacement radiographically.

Intrusive luxation

In intrusive luxation, tooth is forced into its socket in an apical direction. It is most damaging injury to a tooth particularly for pulp and the supporting structures. When examined clinically, the tooth is in infraocclusion, on percussion metallic sound is heard. In mixed dentition, diagnosis is more difficult as intrusion can mimic a tooth undergoing eruption.

Pulp

It is a soft tissue of mesenchymal origin residing within the pulp chamber and root canals of teeth.

Bleaching

It is a procedure which involves lightening of the color of a tooth through the application of a chemical agent to oxidize the organic pigmentation in the tooth.

Closed chamber bleaching/extracoronal bleaching

In this technique, instead of removing the existing restoration, the bleaching paste is applied to the tooth via bleaching tray.

Resorption

A condition associated with either a physiologic or a pathologic process resulting in the loss of dentin, cementum or bone.

Root-resorption

An unusual form of tooth resorption that begins centrally within the tooth, apparently initiated in most cases by a peculiar inflammation of the pulp. It is characterized by oval shaped enlargement of root canal space.

Internal inflammatory resorption

A type of internal resorption in which progressive loss of dentin is present without the deposition of any form of hard tissue in the resorption cavity.

External root resorption

This type of resorption is initiated in the periodontium and it affects the external or lateral surface of the root.

Surface resorption

A transient phenomenon in which the root surface undergoes spontaneous destruction and repair. It is the least destructive form of external root résorption. It is a self-limiting process; hence, it requires no treatment.

Cervical root resorption (extracanal invasive resorption)

The type of inflammatory root resorption occurring immediately below the epithelial attachment of tooth. Epithelial attachment need not be always exactly at the cervical margin but can also be apical to the cervical margin.

Tooth infraction

Incomplete tooth fracture extending partially through a tooth. The fracture commonly involves enamel and dentin,while, sometimes pulp and periodontal structure in few cases.

Vertical root fracture

A longitudinally oriented fracture of root that originates from the apex of tooth and progresses to the coronal part of tooth.

Dentin hypersensitivity

A sharp, short pain arising from exposed dentin in response to stimuli typically thermal, chemical, tactile or osmotic and which cannot be ascribed to any other form of dental defect or pathology.

Indirect pulp capping

It is a procedure performed in a tooth with deep carious lesion adjacent to the pulp. In this procedure, caries near the pulp is left in place to avoid pulp exposure and is covered with a biocompatible material.

Direct pulp capping

This procedure involves the placement of biocompatible material over the site of pulp exposure to maintain vitality and promote healing.

Pulpotomy

It refers to coronal extirpation of vital pulp tissue.

Partial pulpotomy

It implies removal of the coronal pulp tissue upto the level of healthy pulp. Calcium hydroxide is material of choice for pulpotomy in young permanent teeth to stimulate the formation of dentine bridge in cariously exposed pulp.

Cervical or complete pulpotomy

It involves removal of entire coronal pulp to the level of root orifices. It is performed when pulp is inflamed to deeper levels of coronal pulp.

Formocresol pulpotomy

It is reparative, devitilizing and popular pediatric pulp therapy advocated by Sweet in 1930.

Apexification

Apexification is the process of inducing the development of the root and the apical closure in an immature pulpless tooth with an open apex. It is different from apexogenesis, in that,in later root development occurs by physiological process.

Lasers

It is an acronym for Light Amplification by Stimulated Emission of Radiation. The application of lasers is almost in every field of human endeavor from medicine, science and technology to business and entertainment over the past few years.

Endoscope

Endoscope offers a better magnification than loupes or a microscope. It is mainly used during surgical endodontic treatment.

Orascope

Orascope is a fiber optic endoscope. It is mainly used for intracanal fibers. Quality of image produced by orascope is directly related to number of fibers.

Classifications

Classifications of Pulpal Pathologies

❑ Baume's Classification
- Based on clinical symptoms:
    - Asymptomatic, vital pulp which has been injured or involved by deep caries for which pulp capping may be done
    - Pulp with history of pain which is amenable to pharmacotherapy
    - Pulp indicated for extirpation and immediate root filling
    - Necrosed pulp involving infection of radicular dentin accessible to antiseptic root canal therapy.

❑ Seltzer and Bender's Classification
- Based on clinical tests and histological diagnosis:
    - Treatable without pulp extirpation and endodontic treatment
        - Intact uninflamed pulp
        - Transition stage
        - Atrophic pulp
        - Acute pulpitis
        - Chronic partial pulpitis without necrosis.
    - Untreatable without pulp extirpation and endodontic treatment

- Chronic partial pulpitis with necrosis
- Chronic total pulpitis
- Total pulp necrosis.

❑ Ingle's Classification
- Inflammatory Changes:
  o Hyperreactive pulpalgia
    - Hypersensitivity
    - Hyperemia.
  o Acute pulpalgia
    - Incipient
    - Moderate
    - Advanced.
  o Chronic pulpalgia
  o Hyperplastic pulpitis
  o Pulp necrosis.
- Retrogressive Changes:
  o Atrophic papulosis
  o Calcific papulosis.

❑ Grossman's Clinical Classification
- Pulpitis:
  o Reversible papulosis
    - Symptomatic (Acute)
    - Asymptomatic (Chronic).
  o Irreversible pulpitis:
    - Acute
      ➤ Abnormally responsive to cold
      ➤ Abnormally responsive to heat.
    - Chronic
      ➤ Asymptomatic with pulp exposure
      ➤ Hyperplastic pulpitis
      ➤ Internal resorption.
- Pulp degeneration:
  o Calcific (Radiographic diagnosis)
  o Other (Histopathological diagnosis).
- Necrosis.

Classifications of Periradicular Pathologies

❑ Grossman's Classification
- Acute periradicular disease:
  - Acute apical periodontitis
    - Vital
    - Nonvital.
  - Acute alveolar abscess
  - Phoenix abscess.
- Chronic periradicular disease with areas of rarefaction:
  - Chronic apical periodontitis
    - Chronic alveolar abscess
    - Periapical granuloma
    - Cystic apical periodontitis.
  - Persistent apical periodontitis
- Condensing osteitis
- External root resorption
- Disease of the periradicular tissues of nonendodontic origin.

❑ WHO Classification

K 04.4	Acute apical periodontitis
K 04.5	Chronic apical periodontitis (apical granuloma)
K 04.6	Periapical abscess with sinus
K 04.60	Periapical abscess with sinus to maxillary antrum
K 04.61	Periapical abscess with sinus to nasal cavity
K 04.62	Periapical abscess with sinus to oral cavity
K 04.63	Periapical abscess with sinus to skin
K 04.7	Periapical abscess without sinus
K 04.8	Radicular cyst (periapical cyst)
K 04.80	Apical and lateral cyst
K 04.81	Residual cyst
K04.82	Inflammatory paradental cyst

❑ Ingle's Classification of Pulpoperiapical Pathosis
  • Painful pulpoperiapical pathosis:
    o Acute apical periodontitis
    o Advanced apical periodontitis
      – Acute apical abscess
      – Phoenix abscess
      – Suppurative apical periodontitis (chronic apical abscess).
  • Nonpainful pulpoperiapical pathosis:
    o Condensing osteitis
    o Chronic apical periodontitis both incipient and advanced stages
    o Chronic apical periodontitis
      – Periapical granuloma
      – Apical cyst
      – Suppurative apical periodontitis.

Nonspecific Mediators of Periradicular Lesions

❑ Nonspecific mediators can be classified into following types
  • Cell derived mediators:
    o Neuropeptides
    o Eicosanoids/arachidonic acid derivatives
    o Cytokines
    o Lysosomal enzymes
    o Platelet activating factor
    o Vasoactive amines
    o Prostaglandins.
  • Plasma derived mediators:
    o Fibrinolytic system
    o Complement system
    o Kinin system.
  • Extracellular matrix derived mediators
  • Effector molecules.

Classification of Sterilization Instruments

Category	Definition	Examples
Critical	Where instruments enter or penetrate into sterile tissue, cavity or blood stream	• Surgical blades and instruments • Surgical dental bur
Semicritical	Which contact intact mucosa or nonintact skin	• Amalgam condenser • Dental handpieces • Mouth mirror • Saliva ejectors
Noncritical	Which contact intact skin	• Pulse oximeter • Stethoscope • Light switches • Dental chair

Classification of Local Anesthetic Agents

❑ Based on chemical structure
- Ester group:
    o Cocaine
    o Benzocaine
    o Procaine
    o Tetracaine.
- Amide (Nonester group):
    o Lidocaine
    o Mepivacaine
    o Prilocaine
    o Etidocaine
    o Bupivacaine.

❑ Based on duration of action
- Short acting:
    o Procaine.
- Intermediate acting:
    o Lidocaine.

- Long acting:
  - Bupivacaine.

Classification of Antibiotics

❑ Based on spectrum of activity

Narrow spectrum	Broad spectrum
Penicillin G	Tetracyclines
Streptomycin	Chloramphenicol
Erythromycin	

❑ Type of action
- Bactericidal:
  - Penicillin and cephalosporins
  - Metronidazole
  - Fluoroquinolone:
    - Nalidixic acid
    - Ciprofloxacin
    - Ofloxacin
    - Sparfloxacin
    - Gatifloxacin.
  - Aminoglycosides:
    - Streptomycin
    - Amikacin.
- Primarily bacteriostatic:
  - Sulfonamides
  - Tetracycline
  - Clindamycin
  - Erythromycin.

❑ On the basis of family
- Penicillins
- Cephalosporins
- Sulfonamides
- Tetracyclines

- Aminoglycosides
- Macrolides.

Classifications of Endodontic Instruments

❑ ISO-FDI (Federation Dentaire International) grouped root canal instruments according to their method of use

Group I	Hand use only, for example, K and H-files, reamers, broaches, etc.
Group II	Latch type engine driven-same design as group I but can be attached to hand piece, e.g., profiles, light speed
Group III	Drills or reamers latch type engine driven, e.g., Gates-Glidden, Peeso reamers
Group IV	Root canal points like gutta percha, silver point, paper point

❑ Grossman's classification

Function	Instruments
Exploring	Smooth broaches and endodontic explorers (to locate canal orifices and determine patency of root canal)
Debriding or extirpating	Barbed broaches (to extirpate the pulp and other foreign materials from the root canal)
Cleaning and shaping	Reamers and files (used to shape the canal space)
Obturating	Pluggers, spreaders and lentulospirals (to pack gutta percha points into the root canal space)

❑ According to method of use
- Group I: Hand-operated endodontic instruments
  - Example: Broaches, files, reamers.
- Group II: Nonrotary endodontic instruments
  - Engine driven instruments:
    - Reciprocating or quarter turn motion

- Vertical stroke along with quarter turn motion.
  - o Ultrasonic and sonic instruments.
- Group III: Rotary endodontic instruments used with a handpiece
  - o Slow speed rotary stainless steel instruments
  - o NiTi rotary instruments.

Classifications of Sealers

❑ According to their composition
- Eugenol
- Noneugenol
- Medicated
- Eugenol containing sealers:
  - o Silver containing cements:
    - Kerr sealer (Rickert, 1931)
    - Procosol radaiopaque silver cement (Grossman, 1936).
  - o Silver free cements:
    - Procosol nonstaining cement (Grossman, 1958)
    - Grossman's sealer (Grossman, 1974)
    - Tubliseal (Kerr, 1961)
    - Wach's paste (Wach).
- Noneugenol:
  - o Diaket
  - o AH-26
  - o Chloropercha and eucapercha
  - o Nogenol
  - o Hydron
  - o Endofil
  - o Glass ionomer
  - o Polycarboxylate
  - o Calcium phosphate cement.
- Medicated:

- o Diaket-A
- o N2
- o Endomethasone
- o SPAD
- o Iodoform paste
- o Riebler's paste
- o Mynol cement
- o Ca(OH)2 paste.
- ❑ According to Grossman
  - Zinc oxide resin cement
  - Calcium hydroxide cements
  - Paraformaldehyde cements
  - Pastes.
- ❑ According to Cohen, ADA specification number 57 classifies endodontic filling materials as follows:
  - Type I, Material intended to be used with core material. It is further classified into three classes:
    - o Class 1: Includes materials in the form of powder and liquid that set through a nonpolymerizing process
    - o Class 2: Includes material in the form of two pastes that sets through a nonpolymerizing process
    - o Class 3: Includes polymers and resin systems that set through polymerization.
  - Type II, Material intended to be used with or without core material or sealer. It is further classified into four classes:
    - o Class 1: Powder and liquid nonpolymerizing
    - o Class 2: Paste and paste nonpolymerizing
    - o Class 3: Metal amalgams
    - o Class 4: Polymer and resin systems polymerization.
- ❑ According to Ingle
  - Cements

- Pastes
- Plastics.
❑ According to Clark
- Absorbable
- Nonabsorbable.
❑ According to Harty FJ
- Pastes and cements may be divided into five groups:
  o Zinc-oxide eugenol based
  o Resin based
  o Gutta percha based cements consists of solutions of gutta percha in organic solvents. Examples; Chloropercha, Eupercha
  o Dentin adhesive materials, e.g., cyanoacrylate cements, glassionomer cements, polycarboxylate cements, calcium phosphate, composite materials.
  o Materials to which medicaments have been added:
    - Those in which strong disinfectants have been added in order to decrease possible postoperative pain, like paraformaldehyde and corticosteroid preparation
    - Those in which calcium hydroxide has been added with the purpose of inducing cementogenesis and dentinogenesis at the foramen, thus creating a permanent biological seal. For examples, calcibiotic root canal sealer (CRCS), sealapex and biocalex.
❑ Methacrylate resin-based sealers:
- First generation methacrylate resin based sealer, e.g., hydron
- Second generation methacrylate resin based sealer, e.g., EndoReEZ
- Third generation methacrylate resin based sealer, e.g., epiphany
- Fourth generation methacrylate resin based sealer, e.g., MetaSEAL, RealSEAL.

Classifications of Endodontic-Periodontal Lesions

❑ According to Weine
  • Based on etiology and treatment plan:
    o Class I: Tooth which clinically and radiographically simulates the periodontal involvement but it is due to pulpal inflammation or necrosis
    o Class II: Tooth has both pulpal and periodontal disease occurring concomitantly
    o Class III: Tooth has no pulpal problem but requires endodontic therapy plus root amputation for periodontal healing
    o Class IV: Tooth that clinically and radiographically simulates pulpal or periapical disease but has periodontal disease.
❑ According to Simon et al (1972)
  • Based on etiology, diagnosis, prognosis and treatment:
    o Type 1: Primary endodontic lesion
    o Type 2: Primary endodontic lesion with secondary periodontal involvement
    o Type 3: Primary periodontal lesions
    o Type 4: Primary periodontal lesion with secondary endodontic involvement
    o Type 5: True combined lesion.
❑ According to Grossman (1988)
  • Oliet and Pollock's classification based on treatment protocol:
    o Type I: Lesions requiring endodontic treatment only. For example:
      – Tooth with necrotic pulp reaching periodontium
      – Root perforations
      – Root fractures
      – Chronic periapical abscess with sinus tract
      – Replants

- Transplants
- Teeth requiring hemisection.
- o Type II: Lesion that require periodontal treatment only. For example;
    - Occlusal trauma causing reversible pulpitis
    - Suprabony or infrabony pockets caused during periodontal treatment resulting in pulpal inflammation
    - Occlusal trauma and gingival inflammation resulting in pocket formation.
- o Type III: Lesions that require combined endodontic and periodontal treatment.
    - Any lesion of type I which result in irreversible reaction to periodontium requiring periodontal treatment
    - Any lesion of type II which results in irreversible damage to pulp tissue requiring endodontic therapy.

Classification of Post

❑ According to Shape
- Parallel-sided–serrated and vented, e.g., parapost
- Tapered self-threading systems, e.g., dentatus
- Tapered smooth-sided systems, e.g., kerr, ash
- Parallel-sided and threaded post-systems, e.g., radix, anchor, kurer anchor post system
- Parallel-sided, threaded and split shank systems, e.g., flexipost.

❑ According to Method of Engagement of Dentin
- Passive (Cemented) Retention Posts:
    - o Cast posts
    - o Smooth tapered
    - o Serrated parallel posts.

❑ Active (Threaded) Retention Posts

- Flexiposts
- Kurer Anchor posts.
❏ According to Material of the Post
- Metal:
  o Stainless steel
  o Titanium
  o Ni-Cr
  o Gold alloy.
- Fiber Posts:
  o Glass fiber
  o Quartz fiber
  o Carbon fiber, e.g.,:
    - Composipost
    - Carbonite
    - Endopost
    - Mirafit carbon.
  o Silicon fiber, e.g.,:
    - Esthetipost
    - Esthetiplus
    - Lightpost
    - Snowpost
    - Parapost fiber white
    - Fiber-kor.
- Ceramic:
  o Ceramic, e.g., compost
  o Zirconia.
- Core.

Classifications of Dentofacial Injuries

❏ The currently recommended classification is one based on the WHO and modified by JO Andreasen and FM Andreasen. This classification is used by International Association of Dental Traumatology.
- Soft tissues

N873.69	Lacerations
N902.0	Contusion
N910.0	Abrasions

- Tooth Fractures

N873.60	Enamel fracture
N873.61	Crown-fractures-uncomplicated (no pulp exposure)
N873.62	Crown-fractures-complicated (with pulp exposure)
N873.64	Crown-root fractures
N873.63	Root fractures

- Luxation Injuries

873.66	Tooth concussion
873.66	Subluxation
873.66	Extrusive luxation
873.66	Lateral luxation
873.67	Intrusive luxation
873.68	Avulsion

- Facial Skeletal Injuries

802.20	Fracture of alveolar process of mandible
802.40	Fracture of alveolar process of maxilla
802.21	Fracture of body of mandible
802.41	Fracture of body of maxilla

❏ Ingle's Classification
- Soft Tissue Injury:
  - Laceration
  - Abrasion
  - Contusion.

- Luxation Injury:
  o Concussion
  o Intrusive luxation
  o Lateral luxation
  o Extrusive luxation
  o Avulsion.
- Tooth Fractures:
  o Enamel fractures
  o Uncomplicated crown fracture
  o Complicated crown fracture
  o Crown-root fracture
  o Root fracture.
- Facial Skeletal Injury:
  o Alveolar process
  o Body of mandible
  o TMJ.

❏ **Ellis and Davey's Classifications (1960)**

Class I	Simple fracture of the crown involving enamel
Class II	Extensive fracture of the crown, with considerable amount of dentin involved but no pulp exposure
Class III	Extensive fracture of the crown, with considerable amount of dentin involved, with pulp exposure
Class IV	Traumatized tooth becomes nonvital (with or without loss of crown structure)
Class V	Tooth lost due to trauma
Class VI	Fracture of root with or without crown or root structure

Contd.

Contd.

Class VII	Displacement of the tooth without crown or root fracture
Class VIII	Fracture of crown en masse
Class IX	Fracture of deciduous teeth

❑ Heitherasy and Marde recommended a classification of subgingival fracture based on level of tooth fracture in relation to various horizontal planes of periodontium, as follows:

Class I	Fracture line does not extend below level of attached gingiva
Class II	Fracture line extends below attached gingiva but not below level of alveolar crest
Class III	Fracture line extends below level of alveolar crest
Class IV	Fracture line is within coronal third of root but below level of alveolar crest

❑ WHO Classification: The following classification was given in 1978 with code no. corresponding to International Classification of Diseases.

873.60	Enamel fracture
873.62	Crown fracture with pulpal involvement
873.63	Root fracture
873.64	Crown-root fracture
873.66	Luxation
873.67	Intrusion or extrusion

Contd.

Contd.

873.68	Avulsion
873.69:	Other injuries such as soft tissue lacerations.
873.61	Crown fracture involving enamel, dentin without pulpal involvement

❏ The following classification was modified by Andreasen:

873.64	Uncomplicated crown–root fracture without pulp exposure
873.64	Complicated crown–root fracture without pulp exposure
873.66	Concussion: Injury to tooth supporting structure without loosening or displacement of tooth
873.66	Subluxation: An injury to tooth supporting with abnormal loosening but without displacement of tooth
873.66	Lateral luxation: Displacement of tooth in a direction other than maxillary and accompanied by fracture of alveolar socket

▌Classification of Cracked Teeth

❏ Cracked teeth can be classified on the basis of pulpal or periodontal involvement and the extent of crack:
  - Class A: Crack involving enamel and dentin but not pulp
  - Class B: Crack involving pulp but not periodontal apparatus
  - Class C: Crack extending to pulp and involving periodontal apparatus

- Class D: Complete division of tooth with pulpal and periodontal apparatus involvement
- Class E: Apically induced fracture.

❏ Two classic patterns of crack formation exist:
- The first occurs when the crack is centrally located, and following the dentinal tubules may extend to the pulp
- The second is where the crack is more peripherally directed and may result in cuspal fracture.

Classification of Laser

❏ According to ANSI and OHSA standards lasers are classified as:

Class I	These are low powered lasers that are safe to use, e.g., Laser beam pointer
Class II	Low powered visible lasers that are hazardous only when viewed directly for longer than 1000 seconds, e.g., He–Ne lasers
Class IIb	Low powered visible lasers that are hazardous when viewed for more than 0.25 seconds
Class IIIa	Medium powered lasers that are normally hazardous if viewed for less than 0.25 seconds without magnifying optics
Class IIIb	Medium powered lasers that can be hazardous if viewed directly
Class IV	These are high powered lasers (>0.5 W) that produce ocular skin and fire hazards

❏ Based on the wavelength of the beam:
- Ultraviolet rays: 140–400 nm
- Visible light: 400–700 nm
- Infrared: 700 to microwave spectrum.

❏ Based on penetration power of beam:
- Hard: Increased penetration power

        o For example, Nd: YAG, argon.
- Soft lasers: Decreased penetration power.
  - For example, diode, Gallium-Sa, He-Ne lasers.
❑ Based on pulsing:
- Pulsed: The beam is not continuous and lasts for short duration.
- Nonpulsed: The beam is continuous with fixed duration.
❑ According to type of laser material used:
- Gas lasers: CO_2 lasers, Argon lasers, He-Ne lasers
- Liquid lasers: Ions of rare earth or organic fluorescent dyes are dissolved in a liquid, e.g., dye lasers.
- Solid state lasers:
  - Ruby lasers
  - Nd: YAG lasers.
- Semiconductor lasers:
  - Gallium
  - Arsenide.

Components of Periodontal Ligament

❑ Periodontal fibers
❑ Cells
❑ Blood vessels
❑ Nerves.

Types of Chronic Pulpitis

❑ Ulcerative/open form
❑ Hyperplastic form
❑ Closed form.

Types of Endodontic Biofilm

❑ Types of endodontic biofilm
- Intracanal biofilms
- Extraradicular biofilms
- Periapical biofilms.

Rubber Dam

- ❑ Rubber dam equipment:
  - Rubber dam sheet
  - Rubber dam clamps
  - Rubber dam forceps
  - Rubber dam frame
  - Rubber dam punch.
- ❑ Rubber dam accessories:
  - Lubricant/petroleum jelly
  - Dental floss
  - Rubber dam napkin.
- ❑ Thickness of rubber dam sheet:

Thin	0.15 mm
Medium	0.20 mm
Heavy	0.25 mm
Extra heavy	0.30 mm
Special heavy	0.35 mm

Classification of Sutures

- ❑ According to absorbency:
  - Absorbable
  - Nonabsorbable.
- ❑ According to physical property:
  - Monofilament
  - Multifilament
  - Twisted or braided.

Discoloration

- ❑ Types of discoloration:
  - Intrinsic discoloration
  - Extrinsic discoloration
  - Combination of both.

❑ Etiology of tooth discoloration:
- Intrinsic stains
  - Pre-eruptive causes:
    - Diseases:
      - Alkaptonuria
      - Hematological disorders
      - Disease of enamel and dentin
      - Liver diseases.
    - Medications:
      - Tetracycline stains and other antibiotic use
      - Fluorosis stain.
  - Posteruptive causes of discoloration:
    - Pulpal changes
    - Trauma
    - Dentin hypercalcification
    - Dental caries
    - Restorative materials and operative procedures
    - Aging
    - Functional and parafunctional changes.
- Extrinsic stains
  - Daily acquired stains:
    - Plaque
    - Food and beverages
    - Tobacco use
    - Poor oral hygiene
    - Swimmer's calculus
    - Gingival hemorrhage.
  - Chemicals:
    - Chlorhexidine
    - Metallic stains.

Classification of Extrinsic Stains (Nathoo in 1997)

❑ N1 type dental stain (direct dental stain): Colored materials bind to the tooth surface to cause discoloration. Tooth has same color, as that of chromogen

❑ N2 type dental stain (direct dental stain): Chromogen changes color after binding to the tooth
❑ N3 type dental stain (indirect dental stain): Prechromogen (colorless) binds to the tooth and undergoes a chemical reaction to cause a stain.

Classifications of Tooth Resorption

❑ Lindskog classification of tooth resorption:
- Physiologic tooth resorption: Seen in deciduous teeth during eruption of permanent teeth
- Pathologic tooth resorption: Seen in both deciduous as well as permanent teeth due to underlying pathology.

❑ Andreasen classification of tooth resorption
- Internal resorption:
  - Root canal replacement resorption
  - Internal inflammatory resorption.
- External resorption:
  - Surface resorption
  - Inflammatory resorption
  - Replacement resorption
  - Dentoalveolar ankylosis.

External Resorption

❑ External resorption is of three types:
- Surface resorption
- External inflammatory root resorption
- Replacement resorption.

❑ On the basis of the location:
- Cervical
- Lateral
- Apical.

❑ It may be found in the following conditions:
- Periodontal disease
- Luxation injuries

- Hypoparathyroidism
- Hyperparathyroidism
- Turner's syndrome
- Paget's disease
- Gaucher's disease
- Radiation therapy.

Viva-Voce

1. **What is the main objective of operative and restorative dentistry?**

Ans: To restore and maintain health of natural dentition

2. **Which is the oldest and most widely used method of tooth nomenclature?**

Ans: Palmer system

3. **Which root canal of the upper first molar would you expect to be most difficult to prepare for root filling?**

Ans: Mesiobuccal

4. **According to FDI system, which tooth is designated number '46'?**

Ans: Permanent mandibular right first molar

5. **Excessive hemorrhage during apical surgery is controlled by**

Ans: Placing epinephrine containing solution in surgical site

6. Teeth most commonly congenitally absent are

Ans: Mandibular 2nd bicuspids

7. The central parts of the temporomandibular joints are

Ans: Avascular without sensory nerve supply

8. The end point of mandibular closure with maximum intercuspation of the teeth is known as

Ans: Centric occlusion

9. Centric relation refers to a

Ans: Retrusive movement

10. The movement which occurs in centric relation is about

Ans: 25 mm

11. Diagnosis of cracked tooth syndrome is made by

Ans: Biting on solid object and release of pressure

12. Most commonly fractured cusp is

Ans: Lingual cusps of mandibular molars

13. "Double inverted cone" type of penetration of dental caries is seen in

Ans: Smooth surface caries

14. Pit and fissure lesions are represented by

Ans: Base of cone facing each other

15. Which is the common site for proximal carious lesions

Ans: Just cervical to contact area

16. In which condition is the salivary duct occluded?

Ans: Sialolithiasis

17. Smooth surface caries is mainly caused by

Ans: *Streptococcus mutans*

18. Patients with which salivary levels of *Streptococcus mutans* are considered at high-risk for dental caries?

Ans: Above 106 CFU/ml

19. A patient with less than 104 CFU of lactobacilli per ml of saliva is associated with

Ans: Low caries risk group

20. The first anti-gingivitis oral rinse approved by FDA and ADA Council is

Ans: 0.12% chlorhexidine gluconate

21. The method of choice for removal of interproximal plaque is

Ans: Multitufted waxed floss

22. Percentage of pit and fissure caries in children is

Ans: 80–90%

23. Incidence of dental caries in young children is most effectively reduced by

Ans: Sealants

24. Remineralization of the cariously damaged tooth structure occurs as local pH

Ans: Rises above 5.5

25. **The term 'odontopathic' refers to:**

Ans: Causing disease to teeth

26. **The term "aciduric" refers to**

Ans: Bacteria capable of tolerating acidic environment

27. **The microorganisms most strongly associated with onset of caries and active progression of cavitated lesions are**

Ans: *Streptococcus mutans* and *lactobacilli*

28. **Nonspecific plaque hypothesis assumes that**

Ans: All plaque are pathogenic

29. **The single most important factor in producing cariogenic plaque is**

Ans: High frequency of sucrose exposure

30. **The teeth normally have a plaque community dominated by**

Ans: *Streptococcus sanguis* and *Streptococcus mitis*

31. **The process of plaque regrowth after the tooth surface is cleaned is termed as**

Ans: Secondary succession of plaque growth

32. **Going from higher to lower demineralization of enamel starts at the pH range from**

Ans: 5–5.5

33. **The second most susceptible area of tooth to caries are**

Ans: Proximal surface gingival to contact area

34. Root caries is initiated by

Ans: *A.viscosus*

35. The time for progression from incipient caries to clinical caries, i.e., cavitation on smooth surfaces is estimated to be

Ans: 18 months ± 6 months

36. What is the difference between white spot of hypocalcification and white spot of incipient caries?

Ans: Incipient caries spot partially or totally disappears visually when hydrated while hypocalcified spot is unaffected on hydration

37. The zone of enamel caries, which is relatively unaffected by caries attack is

Ans: The surface zone

38. Which part of tooth is least resistant to caries?

Ans: Dentinoenamel junction

39. Most effective treatment in preventing pit and fissure caries is

Ans: Pit and fissure sealants

40. Occlusal surfaces account for only of all tooth surfaces

Ans: 12.5%

41. The levels of which bacteria can be used to assess the effectiveness of caries control procedures?

Ans: Lactobacilli

42. **Senile caries is**

Ans: Root surface caries

43. **Dental caries is said to be 'extensive' when**

Ans: Distance between infected dentin and pulp is less than 1mm

44. **A bacteria not associated with caries process is**

Ans: *Staphylococcus aureus*

45. **When ages are equal, studies have shown that young girls have slightly higher caries index than boys. This is attributed to**

Ans: Earlier eruption of dentition in girls

46. **Clinically the earliest evidence of caries is**

Ans: Chalky white area on the tooth

47. **Fluoride-richness of surface enamel**

Ans: Increases with age

48. **A person suffering from xerostomia is more likely to have**

Ans: Increase in lesions of dental caries

49. **Give one contraindication of pit and fissure sealants?**

Ans: They are not used in cavitated lesion

50. **The most reliable index for dentinal caries removal is**

Ans: Tactile stimuli

51. **Caries control is an intermediate step in restorative treatment and most frequently used materials are**

Ans: Amalgam and intermediate restorative material

52. Complete mouth examination requires how many radiographs?

Ans: 4 bitewing and 18 periapical films

53. In panoramic radiography, there is usually overlapping in

Ans: Bicuspid area

54. An accepted solvent for gutta percha is

Ans: Eucalyptol

55. Which instrument is not considered as dental equipment?

Ans: Excavators

56. What is considered the most universal operating position for operator?

Ans: 11 o'clock

57. A common fault in operating at 12 o'clock position is

Ans: Using direct vision and bending of the back and neck of operator

58. The commonly used mouth mirror sizes are

Ans: No. 2 to No. 5

59. Shade determination is easier during esthetic restoration for

Ans: Modifying tooth color

60. The color matching for composites when done in a dry state, would make the tooth appear

Ans: Lighter than the adjacent teeth

61. **The treatment of choice after root canal treatment on mandibular molar with involvement of bifurcation caries is**

Ans: Bisection

62. **GV Black simply classified cavities as**

Ans: One class of pit and fissure and four classes of smooth surface lesions

63. **Cavities that occur exclusively in posterior teeth are**

Ans: Class II cavities

64. **The classes of cavity which occur both in anterior and posterior teeth are**

Ans: Class I and VI

65. **Removal of deep, pulp encroaching caries should be made using**

Ans: Low rotational speeds

66. **Number of point angles in 'class III' cavity preparation is**

Ans: 3

67. **In order to assume a sound enamel margin, the cavosurface angle of occlusal wall of class V cavity should be**

Ans: 120°–130°

68. **Dr GV Black laid the scientific foundation of cavity preparation in the year**

Ans: 1898

69. **In apicoectomy, a typical surgical flap used**

Ans: Should extend one or two tooth/teeth laterally

70. In "complex" cavity preparation, how many surfaces are involved?

Ans: Three or more surfaces are involved

71. Which is not an internal wall of a cavity preparation?

Ans: Gingival wall

72. Which type of wall is not external wall of a cavity preparation?

Ans: Axial wall

73. A cavity preparation which includes both internal and external cavity walls is termed

Ans: Intracoronal preparation

74. Enameloplasty is indicated

Ans: When fissure depth is not more than 1/3rd thickness of enamel

75. The class V cavity preparation is

Ans: Convex mesiodistally

76. Class V division 1 cavities are

Ans: Cavities on gingival one-third (cervical-third) of facial surfaces of tooth

77. Cavities of the cusp tips of the posterior teeth are

Ans: Class VI cavities

78. Cavities occurring on the lingual fossa of incisors are

Ans: Class I cavities

79. Which wall is the base of class III preparation?

Ans: Axial

80. External outline form of the cavity is influenced by all, except

Ans: Proximity to the pulp

81. Crossing the obligue ridge in maxillary permanent first molar is not permissible

Ans: In incipient caries in mesial and distal pits

82. The wall that is not present in a class V cavity in an anterior tooth is

Ans: Labial wall

83. Gingival wall in a proximal cavity preparation is located

Ans: Apical to the interproximal contact

84. One of the most frequent causes for the failure of the treated pulpless tooth is

Ans: Fracture of the crown

85. Which dental material is contraindicated beneath composite resins as liner/base?

Ans: Zinc oxide-eugenol

86. Who was the first to describe that the mixture of oil of clove and zinc oxide forms a plastic mass and hardens ?

Ans: EC Chisolm

87. Zinc oxide-eugenol liners are

Ans: Bacteriostatic

88. Which dental material does not resist acid-etching?

Ans: Calcium hydroxide

89. **Which cement base has thermal conductivity similar to dentin?**

Ans: Zinc phosphate

90. **Traditionally, zinc phosphate has been the cement base of choice due to**

Ans: High compressive strength and thermal conductivity similar to dentin

91. **Which cements form chemical bond with the tooth structure?**

Ans: Zinc polycarboxylate and glass ionomer

92. **For effective thermal insulation, the minimal thickness of zinc phosphate base should be**

Ans: 0. 75 mm

93. **Cavity varnishes are contraindicated with which two dental materials?**

Ans: Zinc polycarboxylate bases and zinc oxide base

94. **Cavity varnish is indicated under amalgam restorations because it**

Ans: Improves the marginal seal

95. **The best method of increasing the working time of zinc phosphate cement is by**

Ans: Cooling the glass slab used for mixing cement

96. **The consistency of the cements can be quantified by measurement of the**

Ans: Viscosity

97. **The agent used to provide barrier against passage of irritant into the dentinal tubules is**

Ans: Cavity varnish

98. **The cement base materials which have chemical adhesion to tooth structure are**

Ans: Zinc polycarboxylate and glass ionomer

99. **The rationale for placing a liner of glass ionmer cement under a large and deep composite restoration in a molar tooth is**

Ans: Seal the dentinal surface under the composite

100. Iontophoresis helps in

Ans: Reducing dentin sensitivity

101. Which restorative material is most widely used inspite of certain drawbacks?

Ans: Dental amalgam

102. Posterior composite restorations are successful in all of the situations, except

Ans: Moisture is not taken care of

103. The best treatment for class V lesion on a tooth along with extensive class II caries is

Ans: A full crown restoration

104. Ideally, isolation of the operative field is accomplished by use of

Ans: Rubber dam

105. Who was the originator of the rubber dam?

Ans: Dr SC Barnum

106. Dental rubber dam is available in the width of

Ans: 2.5–15 cm

107. What are advantages of dark shade rubber dam?

Ans: It provides good contrast with teeth and it reduces light reflection

108. The six-inch width rubber dam is used with

Ans: Enodon frame and elastic strap

109. Which frames permit the formation of a rubber dam pouch?

Ans: Enodon frame

110. "Theta triangles" refer to

Ans: Absorbent wafers

111. The most effective and widely used acceptable mechanical gingival tissue management during operative procedures is

Ans: Fine cotton fibers with ZnO-eugenol type of cement

112. Which is the most appropriate instrument for removing gutta percha cone from root canal?

Ans: Peeso type reamer

113. The rapid and easy method of tooth separation is

Ans: Mechanical separation

114. Elliot separator works on the principle of

Ans: Wedge

115. Which is the double bow separator?

Ans: Ferrier separator

116. Ferrier double bow separators work on the principle of

Ans: Traction

117. The most common cause of endodontic failure is

Ans: Incomplete obturation

118. Width of the rubber dam for successful use is

Ans: 5 and 6 inches

119. Mineral trioxide aggregate used in apexification

Ans: Dissolves as the apical barrier formation progression

120. The position or manner of use of an instrument is described by

Ans: Suborder

121. Basic instrument formula consists of

Ans: Three digits/units

122. In a three unit formula, the second unit denotes

Ans: Blade length in mm

123. The first unit of basic instrument formula denotes

Ans: Blade width in 1/10 mm

124. The fourth unit added to the basic three unit instrument formula placed at 2nd position denotes

Ans: Angle formed between cutting edge and central axis of the shaft

125. In general sense, all the hand-cutting instruments are

Ans: Excavators

126. The spoon excavator is

Ans: Modified hatchet

127. Which instruments are used for placing retentive grooves for amalgam and composite resins ?

Ans: Small round burs nos. ¼–½

128. For the best results after a root amputation, what is used to seal the apical opening of the canal?

Ans: Gold foil

129. A "chisel" is used to cleave away unsupported proximal enamel and to plane and finish proximal enamel walls with

Ans: Palm and thumb grasp

130. In non-cutting instruments, the part which corresponds to the blade is

Ans: Nib

131. The cutting instrument hoe is subdivision of

Ans: Excavator

132. In an instrument formula, the second number for gingival marginal trimmer is 90–100. The angle former is used on

Ans: Distal gingival margin

133. The most important design characteristic of a 'bur' blade is

Ans: Rake angle

134. For cutting hard and brittle material, which rake angle is needed to increase tool life?

Ans: Negative

135. When using diamond instrument for tooth cutting without coolants, they produce

Ans: More damaging heat as compared to carbide bur

136. Noise level which can cause hearing damage is

Ans: Above 75 db

137. Hand-cutting instruments are made up of

Ans: Carbon stainless steel

138. Cutting edges on carbon steel have

Ans: No protective plating

139. Cutting edges are dulled by

Ans: Contact with hard tooth structures

140. Sharpening is done by

Ans: Arkansas stone

141. Magnifying loupes in the sharpening instruments are useful for

Ans: Evaluating the condition of the cutting edge

142. The approximate maximum speed at which an air turbine hand-piece works is

Ans: 360,000–400,000 rpm

143. The instrument formula numbers placed on the handle are in the following sequence

Ans: Width of the blade, length of the blade, cutting edge angle

144. The type of chisel that has a curved blade is the

Ans: Wedelstaedt chisel

145. The reason for discoloration of pulpless teeth is

Ans: Hemorrhage, decomposition of necrotic pulp, dentin staining drugs, silver nitrate and amalgam

146. Arkansas stone is used for

Ans: Sharpening steel instruments

147. Which ADA specification covers dental amalgam alloy?

Ans: ADA specification no.1

148. The low copper dental amalgam alloy contains maximum amount of copper upto

Ans: 6%

149. Which is the weakest and most corrodible phase of dental amalgam?

Ans: Sn8Hg

150. In high copper dental amalgam alloy, which phase either diminishes or is eliminated?

Ans: 2 phase

151. The 'walking bleach' technique is done by

Ans: Mixture of sodium perborate and 30% hydrogen peroxide

152. From a clinical standpoint, the dental amalgam is

Ans: Insoluble

153. Which material was advertised as the "Royal Mineral Succedaneum" by the Crawcour brothers in United States?

Ans: Restorative resins

154. When a cavity is prepared for silver amalgam, the provision made to prevent displacement of filling is

Ans: Retention form

155. Ideal relationship of the enamel wall and amalgam surface is

Ans: Butt-type junction

156. The outline form of class V amalgam cavity is dictated principally by

Ans: Extension of caries process

157. In class V amalgam cavity the retention grooves are placed in the

Ans: Cervical and occlusal wall

158. When the pulpoaxial line angle in class II cavity preparation is not bevelled/rounded, stress is concentrated in

Ans: Amalgam surrounding line angle

159. Where are the retention grooves for class II amalgam cavity placed in dentin?

Ans: Buccal and lingual proximal wall

160. Which ADA specifications defines the purity of dental mercury?

Ans: ADA specification no.6

161. The triturated mass of amalgam is further worked to enhance the uniformity and plasticity of the mass, the process is called as

Ans: Mulling

162. The most predominant and strongest phase of the amalgam mass is

Ans: Gamma

163. When the diameter of the condenser point reduces to half, the force delivered would be same when applied load is

Ans: Approximately one-fourth of original force

164. Tytin is a

Ans: Rapid reacting dental amalgam alloy

165. According to the survey (1985) of most dentists of Canada and USA, the principal reason behind replacing a restoration was

Ans: Secondary caries

166. Finishing and polishing of amalgam restorations are completed by

Ans: Tin oxide slurry

167. "Rhein trimmers" are instruments which accomplish

Ans: Removal of discrepancies existing in gingival area

168. The isthmus width for class II amalgam cavity should be

Ans: $1/4^{th}$ the intercuspal width

169. While condensing amalgam, a large diameter condenser nib requires

Ans: Greater condensation pressure

170. Condensation time for an amalgam mix is usually

Ans: 3–4 minutes

171. In preparing a Class II amalgam cavity, the proximal box surface has "reverse curve" usually in

Ans: Facial wall

172. In an ideal conservative class II amalgam cavity, the mesiofacial and mesiolingual margins should clear adjacent teeth by

Ans: 0.2–0.3 mm

173. The recommended creep value for amalgam should not, exceed

Ans: 1%

174. If both class II and class V lesions are present on a tooth and they are to be restored by amalgam, then best will be

Ans: Class II preparation and restoration is done followed by class V

175. For amalgam capping, it is mandatory to reduce cusp when facial extension is two-thirds from primary groove toward cusp tip. It provides

Ans: Adequate resistance form

176. Discoloration of the tooth under big amalgam restoration can be prevented by

Ans: Using cavity varnish

177. **The intercuspal width of an ideal class I cavity (occlusal) preparation for amalgam should be**

Ans: 1/4

178. **The amalgam restoration should be burnished after**

Ans: 2–3 minutes

179. **Which is the weakest phase of the set amalgam?**

Ans: Gamma- 2

180. **Delayed expansion of amalgam starts**

Ans: After 3–5 days

181. **Which flap design provides maximum access and visibility?**

Ans: Trapezoidal flap

182. **The minimum strength of amalgam restoration after 1 hour should be**

Ans: Causes delayed expansion of the restoration minimizes the formation of oxides

183. **After few months the marginal leakage in dental amalgam restoration**

Ans: Decreases due to formation of corrosion products

184. **The most common cause for fracture of proximal part of class II amalgam restoration is**

Ans: Improper resistance form of cavity

185. **Which type of amalgam exhibits least creep and marginal breakdown ?**

Ans: High copper spherical alloy

186. Resistance to proximal displacement in a class II amalgam cavity is provided by

Ans: Occlusal dovetail

187. Name the metal in dental amalgam alloy in which mercury would dissolve maximum?

Ans: Tin

188. When does delayed expansion of amalgam start?

Ans: After 3–5 days

189. Gingival cavosurface margin is beveled in a class II cavity for amalgam restoration to

Ans: Remove the unsupported enamel rods

190. How many line angles are found in class II amalgam cavity ?

Ans: 11

191. Which type of pin is most frequently used?

Ans: Self-threading pin

192. What is advantage of placement of pin in amalgam restorations?

Ans: It improves both retention and resistance

193. Most widely used self-threading pin is

Ans: Thread mate system(TMS) pins

194. The least traumatic and most versatile pin system is

Ans: Cemented wire pin

195. The most retentive pin system is

Ans: Self-threading pin

196. For the complex amalgam restorations, Amalgapin technique was developed by

Ans: Shavell

197. In pin-retained amalgam restorations, which property significantly decreases?

Ans: Tensile strength

198. A grossly decayed tooth was restored using self-threading pin. The diameter of pin hole is

Ans: Smaller than diameter of pin

199. The friction-locked pin system described by Goldstein is

Ans: 2–3 times more retentive than cemented pin

200. The optimum pin length in amalgam of a pin-retained restoration is

Ans: 2 mm

201. In pin-retained amalgam restoration, failure is more likely to occur at the

Ans: Pin-dentin interface

202. The optimal depth in dentin for self-threaded pin system is

Ans: 1.5–2 mm

203. Depth of hole of cemented pins should be

Ans: 3–4 mm

204. Friction-locked pins are retained by

Ans: Resiliency of dentin

205. Which pins are used in pulpotomized or root canal treated teeth ?

Ans: Cemented pins

206. Using excessive number of pins in a restoration

Ans: Weakens the restoration

207. In the thread mate system (TMS)

Ans: The pin is slightly oversized

208. The function of pins in large amalgam restoration is to

Ans: Increase retention of amalgam

209. The least microleakage among all dentin pin systems is exhibited by

Ans: Thread mate system system

210. When three or more pinholes are placed in dentin they should be

Ans: At different levels

211. The minimum clearance around the pin for condensation of amalgam is

Ans: 0.5 mm

212. The direction of retentive pinholes should be

Ans: In the direction of long axis of tooth and parallel to nearest external surface

213. The effect of bleaching of vital teeth

Ans: Can initiate cervical erosion response

214. Pin-retained restorations

Ans: Enhances both retention and resistance of restoration

215. The cemented pins were introduced by

Ans: Markley in 1958

216. Luting cements may get rapidly dissolved due to

Ans: Marginal leakage

217. The correct method for diagnosing tetracycline staining is by

Ans: Ultra-violet light

218. Which methods prevent microleakage around porcelain inlay?

Ans: Closer fit and use of dual cure resin cement

219. Finishing of the composite resin is done by

Ans: Fine aluminum oxide and silicon carbide disks

220. With composite resin restoration, finishing of margins is done in sequence of

Ans: Cervical, proximal and occlusal

221. Finishing and polishing of an amalgam restoration is done

Ans: After 24 hours of placing amalgam

222. Over-contoured buccal or lingual surfaces can result in

Ans: Cheek biting

223. Indirect cast gold restorations are primarily finished and polished

Ans: Before casting is tried on tooth

224. Polishing of an amalgam restoration is done best

Ans: After 24 hours

225. The time required for remineralization of dentin after placement of temporary restoration is about

Ans: 8–16 weeks

226. Knoop hardness number of enamel is

Ans: 343

227. Knoop hardness number of dentin is

Ans: 68

228. What is autotransplantation?

Ans: It is the transplantation of a tooth or tooth bud from one socket of one person into the socket of another person of same species

229. After intentional replantation

Ans: Replanted tooth may lead to reattachment without ankylosis

230. The number of dentinal tubules ranges from

Ans: 15,000–20,000/mm^2 at dentinoenamel junction to 45,000–65,000/mm^2 towards pulp

231. The insertion of a tooth in its socket after its complete avulsion is called

Ans: Replantation

232. The prognosis for a tooth with apical resorption is

Ans: Good if the apex can be properly sealed

233. Internal resorption present on primary teeth is treated by

Ans: Pulpectomy

234. Symptoms of internal resorption include

Ans: Completely symptom-free or mild pain at the tolerable level

235. The first translucent filling material produced by Fletcher was

Ans: Silicate cement

236. After setting, the silicate surface exhibits severe crazing and increase in solubility and opacity due to

Ans: Dehydration

237. The basic polymer of the composite resin system was developed by

Ans: Dr Ray Bowen

238. The excellent esthetic restorative material is

Ans: Porcelain

239. The fillers mostly used for composite resin are quartz and lithium aluminum silicate glass because they exhibit

Ans: Chemical inertness

240. Most conventional 'macrofilled' restorative resins contain fillers by weight upto

Ans: 80–90%

241. **The setting reaction for composite resins is free radical polymerization. The initiator of polymerization using visible light is**

Ans: Photosensitive diketone compounds

242. **The surface hardness of composite resins when compared with unfilled resin is**

Ans: Almost twice of unfilled resin

243. **In composite restorative material, the bond present between filler particles and polymer is**

Ans: Silane bond

244. **Internal resorption is least likely to continue in a tooth with**

Ans: A necrotic pulp

245. **Possible contraindications for periapical surgery are**

Ans: The danger of damage to adjacent structures

246. **The most popular resin system in clinical practice is**

Ans: Photo-initiated resin system

247. **For photo-initiated resin system, the optimum depth of cure is obtained with emitting orifice held**

Ans: Within 1 mm of resin surface

248. **When there is no need to support functional stresses, the choice of composite resin in esthetic restoration is**

Ans: Microfilled composite resin

249. A patient comes with esthetic complaint. It was found on examination that teeth are thin labiolingually. The material for maintaining tooth color and contour is

Ans: Hybrid composite resin

250. The esthetic restorative materials minimizing/ reducing the possibility of secondary caries are

Ans: Silicate and glass ionomer cement

251. Currently the most effective agent for removing smear layer while retaining the dentinal plug is

Ans: Polyacrylic acid

252. Occluprint is used for

Ans: Occlusal carving of composite resin class I filling

253. 'Bowen' resin is

Ans: Reaction product of glycidyl methacrylate and bisphenol-A

254. What is Knoop hardness number for composites and Dicor ?

Ans: Composites is 30 and Dicor is 362

255. Which material has lowest coefficient of thermal expansion?

Ans: Dicor 'MGC'

256. Cavity varnishes can be used under all types of restorations, except

Ans: Resins

257. Coefficient of thermal expansion currently available porcelain is

Ans: 14 x 10–6/°Cv

258. Polishable composites refer to

Ans: Microfilled resins

259. Compomer is also known by the terminology

Ans: Polyacid modified composite resin

260. In preparing a class III cavity for restorative resins, the most prominent retention groove is placed within

Ans: Cervical wall

261. The axial wall of the class V cavity preparation is

Ans: Convex

262. Which cavosurface margin is not beveled in class IV cavity preparation for restorative resins?

Ans: Cervical floor

263. A base or liner which is contraindicated beneath filled or unfilled resins is

Ans: Zinc oxide-eugenol

264. The usual sequence of restoration class (type) D depth cavity with composite resin is

Ans: Calcium hydroxide, glass ionomer and filled resin

265. The angle of pulling mylar matrix strip for class III cavity preparation with filled resin is towards

Ans: Incisal direction

266. Beveled cavity design for directly placed composites is most frequently used with

Ans: Class II cavity

267. In restoring class I and class VI cavities with directly placed composites, the cavity design primarily used is

Ans: Modified preparation design

268. The liquid system of glass ionomer restorative material is essentially

Ans: Polyacrylic-itaconic acid

269. An aged patient with high caries index has class III carious lesion extending onto the root surface. Material of choice to restore the carious lesion is

Ans: Glass ionomer cement

270. "Miracle mix" refers to a

Ans: Metal modified glass ionomer cement

271. Concurrent endodontic and periodontic treatment

Ans: May save an apparently hopeless tooth

272. An EBA cement refers to a

Ans Modified zinc oxide-eugenol cement

273. Itaconic acid in the glass ionomer cement liquid

Ans: Inhibit gelation caused by intermolecular hydrogen bonding

274. The setting reaction of glass ionomer cement is basically

Ans: An acid-base reaction

275. The restorative material that is most anticariogenic is

Ans: Glass ionomer cement

276. In preparing a post, the apical root canal seal necessary to prevent leakage is

Ans: Minimum 5–6 mm

277. "Richmond" or Davis crown is

Ans: Post type porcelain crown

278. Fused porcelain jacket crown was developed by

Ans: Dr CH Land

279. The type of crown indicated where both aesthetics and strength are required is

Ans: Porcelain fused to metal crown

280. The core of the aluminous porcelain jacket crown is approximately composed of

Ans: 50% porcelain and 50% alumina

281. Aluminous porcelain jacket crown was developed by

Ans: John McLean

282. Dicor is a

Ans: Castable ceramic restoration

283. Dicor crown was developed by

Ans: Corning Glass Works

284. What is a contraindication for porcelain fused to metal crown?

Ans: Large pulp organ

285. For cementation of porcelain jacket crown with zinc phosphate, the powder for color trial is mixed with

Ans: Glycerine and water solution

286. CEREC system is

Ans: First commercially available CAD/CAM system

287. Major disadvantage of CAD/CAM system is

Ans: Need for extended training and high cost

288. In providing indirect tooth-colored 'onlay', a temporary resin is given. Which cement should be avoided?

Ans: Zinc oxide-eugenol

289. A postoperative alginate impression is a must for temporary resin using

Ans: Indirect temporary technique

290. Acidulated fluorides should not be used in patients with

Ans: Porcelain type crowns

291. While preparing the porcelain inlay cavity the bur should be held

Ans: Parallel to the line of withdrawal

292. In groove and postdesign of an anterior porcelain inlay the groove is placed on

Ans: Axial wall

293. One of the major problems in firing dental porcelain is

Ans: The high degree of shrinkage that occurs

294. Copy milling is related to the

Ans: Fabrication of CAD/CAM restoration

295. 'Command set' refers to dental material that hardens by

Ans: Photo (light) activation

296. Composite restoration may not be fabricated

Ans: By casting using lost wax technique

297. Which American Dental Association specification number covers the 'inlay casting gold'?

Ans: No. 5

298. Majority of cast gold restorations uses

Ans: Type II gold alloys

299. A basic requirement of all cavity preparation for onlay is

Ans: Cavity walls must diverge from floor to occlusal surface

300. Placement of bevels on cavosurface margin for cast gold restorations results in

Ans: 25–35° metal margin

301. In cavity designing for cast gold, the flare of the proximal walls should form axioproximal angles of

Ans: 100°–110°

302. The least costly rubber-based impression material is

Ans: Polysulfides

303. Permissible delay in pouring hydrocolloid impression after removal from mouth is upto

Ans: Half an hour

304. **For proper venting of air and gases, the sprue length is approximately**

Ans: 6–8 mm

305. **The principal retention form for cast metal restoration is**

Ans: Almost parallel vertical walls

306. **'Skirts' are retentive features usually used with**

Ans: Cast gold restoration

307. **The major disadvantage of zinc phosphate cement regarding cementation of a casting is**

Ans: Initially it has a low pH

308. **During cementation of inlay the main problem is**

Ans: If there is an increased mobility in the axial direction

309. **During cementation of onlay the main problem is**

Ans: If there is an increased mobility in the axial direction

310. **What is inlay?**

Ans: Intracoronal restoration fabricated extraorally

311. **The outline form for inlays is**

Ans: Dependent on the extent of destruction

312. **Ideally inlay cavity walls should be**

Ans: Straight and parallel

313. **The factor which contributes maximum for retention of an onlay is**

Ans: Near parallel walls

314. The most critical factor for retaining the casting is

Ans: Taper of walls

315. In inlay preparations the axiopulpal depth should be

Ans: Less in comparison to that of amalgam preparation

316. A cast restoration is maintained in position under masticatory load primarily by virtue of

Ans: The retention and resistance form

317. The outline form for cast restoration is produced by

Ans: Slight tapered fissure bur

318. A gold inlay for class I cavity in a posterior tooth having life expectancy of 10 years in a patient having heavy masticatory force is considered when

Ans: Patient is about 50 years old

319. A secondary flare is given to

Ans: Facial and lingual proximal walls

320. In MOD preparation for gold inlays, gingival bevel should be

Ans: 30°

321. The cavity wall towards the line of withdrawal of wax pattern for inlay should have a taper of

Ans: 2–5°

322. During cusp reduction the reverse (contra) bevel is

Ans: 1/3rd that of inside bevel

323. For gold inlay the occlusal cavosurface bevel is approximately

Ans: 30°–40°

324. To avoid distortion the thickness of rubber base impression material should be

Ans: About 2 mm

325. For maximum accuracy the die from alginate impression should be poured

Ans: Within 30 minutes

326. Inlay waxes used for the direct method procedure possess

Ans: Minimum flow below 37°

327. Inlay wax patterns should be invested as soon as possible in order to minimize change in dimensions caused by

Ans: Relaxation of internal stress

328. An ideal location to attach a sprue pin in a wax pattern is

Ans: Thickest point

329. The initial procedure in fitting a MOD gold inlay casting to a tooth is

Ans: Adjust the contact areas

330. Which procedure removes oxides from the casting

Ans: Pickling

331. The incisal step for class IV cavity for gold type II inlay is indicated

Ans: To arrest attritional wear

332. In inlay preparations the axiopulpal depth in comparison to amalgam should be

Ans: Less

333. **The strength of dental investment for gold alloy is dependent on the amount of**

Ans: Gypsum

334. **Maximum permissible setting expansion of high strength stone is**

Ans: 0.1%

335. **Which is the most biocompatible elastomeric impression materials?**

Ans: Addition silicone

336. **Which dental material shows most tear resistance?**
Ans: Polyether

337. **Crucible indicated for casting-base metal alloys is**

Ans: Quartz crucible

338. **Name few passivating alloys ?**

Ans: Chromium, gold, titanium

339. **Monophase elastomeric impression materials are based on**

Ans: Regular body

340. **Rheology is the study of**

Ans: Flow of matter

341. **Wet corrosion is an example of**

Ans: Electrochemical corrosion

342. **The most unique feature of Nitinol alloy is its**

Ans: Shape memory

343. Retention of gold inlay is maximized by

Ans: Increasing the axial length of the preparation

344. The property of least importance for a luting cement is

Ans: Strength

345. The region of tooth more challenging to restore with greatest change in 'chroma' is

Ans: Cervical third

346. In indirect veneering, labial surface preparation removes approx. 0.5–1 mm enamel and margins are prepared slightly incisal to free gingival crest with a finish line as

Ans: Chamfer finish line

347. Which material is most popular for indirect veneering technique?

Ans: Feldspathic porcelain

348. A silane primer is used to condition the internal surface of which indirect veneer?

Ans: Porcelain veneer

349. It has been found that direct veneer restorations have more limited prognosis and tendency to discolor within

Ans: 3–5 years

350. Most of the direct filling golds are

Ans: 24 karat

351. Electroloy is

Ans: Mat gold alloyed with calcium and wrapped in gold foil

352. Annealing of direct filling gold is done

Ans: To make it cohesive

353. When restoring a tooth with direct filling gold, the condensation should begin at

Ans: Central area of cavity

354. "Mat foil" is

Ans: Mat gold wrapped in fibrous gold foil

355. The direct filling gold which produces the hardest surface on condensation is

Ans: Mat gold alloyed with calcium and wrapped in gold foil

356. The oldest form of direct filling gold used for restorations are

Ans: Fibrous gold foil

357. Which direct filling gold is used both as bulk filler and for surface restoration?

Ans: Encapsulated powdered gold

358. Total root amputation

Ans: Is a logical procedure when an individual root is hopelessly involved

359. The purpose of adding 'calcium' to mat gold is

Ans: To increase hardness and strength

360. Cavities prepared for direct filling gold are thoroughly cleaned, dried and cavity varnish is applied to

Ans: Only dentin

361. Veneered gold foil restoration is

Ans: Combined use of mat foil and gold foil

362. Direct filling gold is always worked from

Ans: Pulpal line angles towards center of pulpal wall

363. A gold foil no. 3 weighs

Ans: 3 grain

364. Extraply is

Ans: Prerolled thinner no.2 gold foil

365. Which agent is used to prevent the formation of deleterious oxides on gold foil?

Ans: Ammonia

366. If the nib diameter is reduced by half and constant malleting force is given the effective compaction force delivered is

Ans: Four times greater

367. For a class I cavity restored with direct filling gold, restorative phase begins with

Ans: Application of cavity varnish

368. The typical class V cavity design for direct gold filling is

Ans: Trapezoidal

369. In class V direct gold filling cavity, retention is provided by

Ans: Facial convergence of occlusal and gingival walls

370. Polishing of class V direct filling gold restoration is done with

Ans: Fine pumice

371. The property of gold which allows for a better marginal seal is

Ans: Malleability

372. Marginal leakage due to temperature change can occur maximum with

Ans: Unfilled resin

373. The most commonly used type(s) of gold alloy is

Ans: Type II

374. The gold alloys have a melting range of

Ans: 1700–1900°F

375. Platinized gold foil is manufactured by

Ans: Laminating platinum foil between two sheets of gold foil

376. Mat gold is made by

Ans: Electrolytic precipitation

377. Condenser nibs have

Ans: Pyramidal serrations

378. Fine powdered gold wrapped in gold foil is known as

Ans: Goldent

379. Degassing of Goldent is done by

Ans: Heating on mica table over an ethanol flame

380. Direct gold fillings are contraindicated in

Ans: Filling of access openings in root canal treated teeth

381. Degassing renders the gold

Ans: Cohesive

382. Most commonly used gold foil is

Ans: No. 4 foil

383. Electroloy is mat gold alloyed with

Ans: Calcium

384. Extraply is a term used for

Ans: Prerolled cylinders of no. 2 or no. 4 foil wrapped around a regular gold rope

385. The malleting force is directed

Ans: 45° to the wall

386. If the nib diameter is reduced by half the compaction force is

Ans: 4 times more

387. For direct gold filling in the class V cavity the axial wall meets the gingival wall

Ans: In acute angle

388. The cavosurface margin for direct gold filling are prepared with

Ans: 30°–40° bevel

389. Direct filling gold is heated prior to its condensation for the purpose of

Ans: Removing surface contaminants

390. The gold used to form bulk of filling is

Ans: Mat gold

391. Cohesion of direct filling gold at room temperature is an example of

Ans: Welding

392. The amount of force required to compact the direct filling gold is influenced most by

Ans: Surface area of condensor

393. A posterior tooth with cusps undermined with caries may achieve maximum masticatory efficiency if restored by

Ans: Cast gold after amalgam filling as a base in undermined areas

394. The type of gold with highest strength to be used in stress bearing areas is

Ans: Electalloy

395. Restorative dentistry with splinting of teeth is indicated when

Ans: Tipped maxillary and mandibular molars cannot be stabilized by occlusal adjustment

396. Pin ledge restorations with minimal contact with the gingival tissues are preferable for splinting

Ans: Anterior tooth

397. If the margins of the preparation accidentally extend apically to the bottom of the epithelial attachment the injured cementum becomes covered by

Ans: Epithelium

398. Avulsed teeth should be stabilized by

Ans: Splinting

399. The term 'idiopathic erosion' means

Ans: Microfractures as cervical area of tooth flexes under heavy loads

400. Class VI cavities are usually

Ans: Abrasion cavities

401. An incipient carious lesion on an interproximal surface is usually located

Ans: Gingival to contact area

402. The incision, chewing and swallowing of food involves

Ans: Both occlusal and neuromuscular guidance

403. Centric stops are those positions where

Ans: Upper lingual and lower buccal cusp of the posterior teeth as well as cusp tips and incisal edges of the opposing teeth make contact

404. The placement of cusps, grooves and ridges in individual restorations must confirm with the

Ans: Mandibular movement and occlusion

405. Tooth contact in centric relation are found more in

Ans: Swallowing

406. In centric occlusion and centric relation there should be

Ans: Even pressure on the central part of disk of the TMJ

407. Raising the bite with encroachment on the inter-occlusal space may result in

Ans: Intrusion of teeth

408. Occlusal stability is maintained by harmony between the

Ans: Structural and neuromuscular components

409. The key to the establishment of an ideal occlusion is the correct location of

Ans: Centric relation

410. Occlusal guidance side is always on the

Ans: Working side

411. The areas for premature contacts in centric relation are the

Ans: Mesial inclines of the maxillary teeth

412. Working side interferences are found on the

Ans: Lingual inclines of the buccal cusps of the maxillary posterior teeth

413. The common site of the fracture of the amalgam restorations are

Ans Mesial marginal ridge

414. Biting forces should be dissipated along

Ans Long axis of the tooth

415. Free way space is also known as

Ans: Inter-occlusal gap

416. Deep overbite causes impingement on the

Ans: Labial aspect of the mandibular incisors and palatal aspect of the maxillary incisors

417. When the lost mandibular 1st molar has not been replaced, then we see

Ans: Mesial and lingual tipping of mandibular second molar

418. Working side interferences are found on the

Ans: Lingual inclines of the buccal cusps of the maxillary posterior teeth

419. The most deleterious side effect of bleaching on non-vital teeth is

Ans: Cervical resorption

420. The in-office non-vital bleaching technique is

Ans: Thermocatalytic technique

421. Bleaching of vital teeth by "In-office technique" is called as

Ans: Power bleach technique

422. Microabrasion techniques for elimination of discoloration of teeth work by

Ans: Removing surface enamel

423. The best material for sedation of dental pulp is

Ans: Zinc oxide-eugenol

424. Historically, Slice preparation refers to

Ans: Placement of extracoronal taper

425. A cast metal restoration which is an intracoronal preparation and covers one or more cusps but not all, is

Ans: Inlay

426. If the gingivo-occlusal height of the vertical wall of the onlay increases, then the occlusal divergence should

Ans: Increase

427. In cavity preparation for cast metal onlay, counterbevel is not placed on

Ans: Facial cusp of maxillary premolars and facial cusp of maxillary 1st molar

428. What is a disadvantage of skirt preparation?

Ans: It increases the display of metal

429. The bevelled margin for gold inlay cavity

Ans: Has no effect on cement liner

430. The cavosurface margin of gold inlay preparation should be

Ans: Bevelled

431. Type IV gold alloy is not suitable for a simple inlay because

Ans: It has poor marginal adaptation

432. The most important function of the dental pulp is

Ans: Formation of the dentin

433. Four root canals are most frequently found in the

Ans: Maxillary first molar

434. Root canal should be filled upto

Ans: Most constricted apical point

435. The greatest curvature is present in which root canal of mandibular 1st molar?

Ans: Mesiobuccal canal

436. Which cell of dental pulp gives rise to several different types of cells ?

Ans: Mesenchymal cell

437. The number and anatomical form of the roots of teeth is determined by

Ans: Hertwig's epithelial sheath

438. The group of teeth which exhibit the least number of anomalies is the

Ans: Maxillary anteriors

439. Anatomically the root canal of the mandibular lateral incisor is

Ans: Wider labiolingually

440. In mandibular first molar, the mesiolingual canal is located below the

Ans: Mesiolingual cusp

441. The anterior tooth most likely to display two canals is:

Ans: Mandibular lateral incisor

442. Which cell is present maximum in dental pulp ?

Ans: Fibroblast

443. The root apex of the maxillary central incisor approaches most closely to

Ans: The labial cortical plate and the nasal fossa

444. Lateral and accessory canals are formed due to

Ans: Break in Hertwig's root sheath

445. What is the main function of plasma cells?

Ans: Antibody-producing

446. Hertwig's root sheath originates from

Ans: Dental epithelium

447. Whar are Korff's fibers?

Ans: The minute rope-like structures present in the pulp

448. Persistent positive cultures from a root canal for long periods indicate

Ans: Poor coronal seal

449. The percentage of gram-positive flora in root canal is

Ans: 60–75%

450. The most common cause of pulpal inflammation is

Ans: Bacteria

451. The frequency of transient bacteremia has been shown to be highest in patients with

Ans: Multiple extractions

452. Lateral perforations are most often seen in

Ans: Mandibular bicuspids

453. What is disadvantage of using corticosteroids as intracanal medicaments ?

Ans: Re- occurence of infection after some time

454. In root canal treatment which drug is most appropriate for antibiotic prophylaxis?

Ans: Penicillin or erythromycin

455. The drug combination most frequently used to treat acute painful dental conditions with accompanied swelling is

Ans: Analgesic and an antibiotic

456. The corticosteroids are used in endodontic practice

Ans: To reduce pulp inflammation

457. Which test helps to differentiate between an apical abscess and a periodontal abscess ?

Ans: Pulp vitality test

458. Tenderness on percussion of a tooth indicates

Ans: Extension of pulpal disease or infection into the periapical area

459. Electric pulp testers most frequently employ which kind of current?

Ans: Low frequency

460. Radiolucent areas appearing over or around the maxillary central apices could be

Ans: A median anterior maxillary cyst

461. Diagnosis of a tooth with exposed vital pulp and an incompletely formed root is made by

Ans: Clinical findings and roentgenographic evidence

462. Electric pulp testing

Ans: Measures the sensory nerve response to irritant of electricity

463. Mobility test is

Ans: The ability to move tooth between two fingers

464. Electric pulp testing is done to

Ans: Differentiate between vital and nonvital pulp

465. The chances of the removal of broken instrument in root canal are good when

Ans: A small piece of instrument is lodged in the bone beyond the apical area

466. A violent response to heat and instant relief to cold is indicative of

Ans: Acute suppurative pulpitis

467. An acute painful inflammation of the pulp characterised by abscess formation upon the surface of or within the pulp is

Ans: Acute suppurative pulpitis

468. An excessive accumulation of blood in the pulp resulting from vascular congestion is

Ans: Hyperaemia

469. Formation of an ulcer on the surface of the pulp in the region of an exposure is

Ans: Chronic ulcerative pulpitis

470. An acute inflammation of the dental pulp characterized by intermittent paroxysm of pain which recently has become continuous and treated by pulpectomy is known as

Ans: Acute serous pulpitis

471. Exposed vital pulp is diagnosed by

Ans: History, radiograph and clinical findings

472. The pain of a tooth which disappears at once when stimulus is removed is characteristic of

Ans: Reversible pulpitis

473. Regardless of stimulus all afferent impulses from the pulp result in sensation of

Ans: Pain

474. Which pulpal condition does not require pulpectomy:

Ans: Reversible hyperaemia

475. Which two conditions of pulp are most closely related to each other

Ans: Acute suppurative pulpitis and acute serous pulpitis

476. Emergency treatment for pulpal hyperaemia is

Ans: Removal of trauma, cleaning the cavity and placing sedative filling

477. In case of pulp necrosis the treatment advised is

Ans: Root canal treatment

478. For the protection of pulp during restorative procedures, the minimum thickness of remaining pulpal dentin should be

Ans: 2 mm

479. Irreversible pulpitis is usually characterised by

Ans: Severe spontaneous continuous pain

480. The earliest change seen in pulp is

Ans: Hyperaemia

481. Arterial hyperaemia can be treated by

Ans: Protection of fractured or eroded crown by sedative dressing after removal of etiological factor

482. Pain on percussion before root canal treatment indicates

Ans: Inflammation of periodontal tissue

483. The treatment advised in case of acute pulpitis is

Ans: Root canal treatment or extraction

484. The smear layer present on dentinal wall acts to prevent pulpal injury by

Ans: Reducing diffusion of toxic substances through tubules

485. An acute apical abscess usually is due to

Ans: Necrotic pulp

486. Infection of the second mandibular molars is most likely to produce swelling of the

Ans: Submandibular space

487. Cementoma (periapical osteofibrosis) is best differentiated from a periapical granuloma by

Ans: Vitality tests

488. The mental foramen may be mistaken with a periapical lesion on a

Ans: Mandibular premolar

489. In primary teeth, pathologic changes in periapical tissue are more apparent

Ans: In furcation area

490. Which oral lesion requires definite diagnosis prior to initiating root canal treatment

Ans: Periapical osteofibrosis

491. If a sinus is associated with chronic periapical infection of a non-vital tooth, besides root canal treatment, specific treatment for the sinus includes

Ans: No active treatment for the sinus

492. A radiolucent area appearing in radiographs between the apices of a vital maxillary lateral incisor and a vital maxillary canine is probably a

Ans: Globulomaxillary cyst

493. The best treatment for an acute apical abscess is

Ans: Root canal treatment

494. 'Trigeminal neuralgia' can be distinguished from dental pain by

Ans: Presence of 'trigger zone'

495. One hypothesis of pain modulation is based upon the inhibitory-excitatory interaction of afferent fiber synapses. This theory is called

Ans: Gate control theory

496. Phantom tooth pain occurs in

Ans: Pulp expirated teeth

497. The apical foramen is located

Ans: At the anatomical apex in about 46% of all teeth

498. The root that most often contains accessory root canals is

Ans: Mesiobuccal root of maxillary first molar

499. The approach to the distobuccal canal in maxillary molar should be from

Ans: Distolingual area

500. In opening of pulp chamber of mandibular incisors the most common error is

Ans: Labial perforation

501. The access preparation for root canal in a maxillary central incisor most resembles with

Ans: Triangle

502. In mandibular premolars two or more canals are present

Ans: In about 10–25% of the cases

503. Emergency treatment in an acute apical abscess is

Ans: Open root canal for drainage and leave open for 1 or 2 days, prescribe antibiotics and analgesic

504. Partial displacement of teeth (class VI) includes

Ans: Intrusion of teeth

505. In the maxillary canine teeth, the greatest root canal diameter is

Ans: Labiolingual

506. The origin of the calcium ions in a calcific bridge over an exposed pulp and covered with calcium hydroxide is the

Ans: Blood stream via the pulp where exposed

507. The objective of doing pulp capping is to

Ans: Preserve the vitality of the entire pulp

508. Success in pulp capping and pulpotomy is greater in

Ans: Molars than anterior teeth

509. Pulp capping and pulpotomy are indicated for

Ans: Vital immature anterior teeth with wide open apices

510. The degree of success rate of pulpotomy in anterior teeth is

Ans: Very unpredictable

511. Apexification in teeth with blunder buss canals and open apices is best done with

Ans: Calcium hydroxide with camphorated monochlorophenol

512. Formocresol pulpotomy is done in which conditions

Ans: Primary teeth free of inflammation or infection

513. Generally the diagnosis of a root fracture is made on the basis of

Ans: Roentgenographic evidence

514. The objective for pulpotomy is to

Ans: Preserve the vitality of the radicular pulp

515. Biomechanical preparation of root canal is done

Ans: In a wet environment with irrigants flooded in the canal

516. Biomechanical preparation of root canal ensures

Ans: Debridement of root canal

517. Recapitulation process is

Ans: Removing the debris with smaller instruments

518. The solution which is most likely to be used for irrigation purpose is

Ans: Sodium hypochlorite

519. From a very fine canal necrosed pulp is removed through

Ans: Small K-type file

520. Instrumentation well-short from the working length of canal results in

Ans: Shelfing or ledging the canal

521. Most important aspect of cleansing and shaping a canal is

Ans: Do not shape or enlarge the canal until the exact working length has been established

522. If an instrument breaks in a canal during treatment, the procedure should be

Ans: Tell the patient immediately and try to remove the broken piece

523. If a small fragment of K-file is broken in the root canal and could not be removed, the best option is to

Ans: Seal the fragment from all around with sealer and gutta percha point in the root canal

524. The correct method for using a root canal H type file is

Ans: Rasping or pulling motion

525. In the pulp cavity hemorrhage can best be removed by using

Ans: Sodium hypochlorite

526. Sodium hypochlorite is an ideal root canal irrigation solution because

Ans: It is a solvent for organic material like pus and necrotic tissue

527. Hemorrhage in the chamber and canals can often be easily controlled with

Ans: Sodium hypochlorite

528. Debridement of pulp cavity is

Ans: Surgical removal of necrotic or mummified non-vital pulp

529. Factors which predispose to over-filling of a root canal include

Ans: Wrong length estimation

530. For the success of root canal treatment the most important step is

Ans: The accurate determination of the length of the root

531. Intracanal medication is indicated for

Ans: Canal cleaning and disinfection

532. Intracanal medication to be used in tooth in which excessive overinstrumentation has been done is

Ans: Corticosteroid antibiotic paste

533. The symptoms of incomplete fracture or split tooth are

Ans: Pain in one quick stab to constant unexplained toothache

534. Best medicament for inter-visit dressing in root canal treatment is

Ans: Paramonochlorophenol

535. In treating a non-vital central incisor in a young child, what is the most important factor in ensuring continued development of closure of the apex

Ans: Placing a thick mix of calcium hydroxide and CMCP at the apex

536. Mummification of the pulp may be indicated for a

Ans: Carious exposure of a non-vital tooth

537. Intracanal medicament

Ans: Should be non-irritating to the periapical tissues

538. Intracanal medicaments are selected on the basis of

Ans: Antimicrobial action and without adverse reaction on peri-apical tissue

539. The intracanal medicament with longer lasting antimicrobial effect is

Ans: Calcium hydroxide

540. The most effective method for disinfection is

Ans: Boiling water bath

541. The type of surgical flap used most often in routine apical surgery is

Ans: Full flap with single releasing incision

542. The cause of persistent positive cultures from a root canal is most frequently the

Ans: Seepage of saliva into the area of operation

543. Ideal root canal filling material should

Ans: Be dimensionally stable

544. The most important requirement of an ideal root canal cement is

Ans: It should make a hermetic seal

545. Iodine in glycerine is used for

Ans: Treating pericementitis to relieve the symptoms and is palliative in nature

546. The primary gutta percha cone must fill the canal tightly in the

Ans: Apical third

547. Warm gutta percha systems are

Ans: 'Obtura' and 'Ultrafil'

548. Free eugenol in root canal sealer cements is significant because it increases

Ans: Cytotoxicity

549. Solvent used along with file to remove gutta percha is

Ans: Chloroform

550. Chairside sterilization of gutta percha points is best done by

Ans: 5.25% solution of sodium hypochlorite

551. The main component of root canal sealers is mostly

Ans: Zinc oxide

552. The disadvantage of gutta percha used as filling material is

Ans: Lack of rigidity in thinner size

553. In primary teeth root canal filling is done by

Ans: Iodoform paste

554. In single rooted tooth ideal length of the post is

Ans: Equal to the length of clinical crown

555. The term 'tug back' is related to

Ans: Fit of the cone in the apical 2 or 3 mm

556. Which aspect of root canal treatment is most important

Ans: Perfect obturation of root canal system

557. Gutta percha is superior over silver cones as a filling material in that it is more

Ans: Compatible with dowel post preparations

558. The type of flap that offers the greatest surgical access and visibility is

Ans: Full flap with double releasing incision

559. Ideal endodontic obturation occurs when

Ans: Patient loses his acute symptoms

560. The main constituents of most of the root canal sealers are

Ans: Zinc oxide and eugenol

561. Treatment of a symptomless under-filled root canal may include

Ans: Periodic observation

562. The cause of failure in root canal treatment most frequently is

Ans: Incomplete filling with poor condensation of the root canal

563. Commonly used gutta percha solvent is

Ans: Chloroform

564. A negative root canal culture

Ans: Should be obtained before filling the canal

565. The root filling material should reach

Ans: Dentino-cemental junction

566. The best apical seal of a straight root canal can be obtained with

Ans: Gutta percha cone with sealer

567. Routine root canal treatment is contraindicated in case of

Ans: Malformed teeth and roots

568. Paraformaldehyde containing root canal cements may be used in

Ans: Temporary pulpotomy procedures in primary teeth

569. Single visit root canal treatment may be successful if tooth is

Ans: Asymptomatic vital tooth

570. The initial priority in treatment of a root fracture is

Ans: Reduction and immobilization

571. In vertical root fractures, chances of success are

Ans: Poor